TRANSPLANTING HOPE

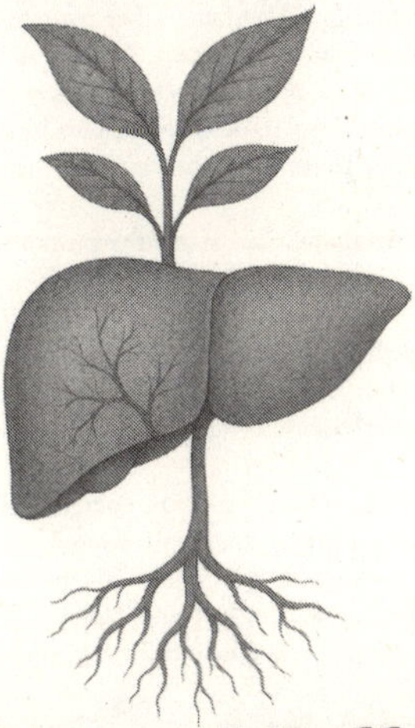

Dr Smita Malhotra
Prof. Anupam Sibal

HarperCollins *Publishers* India

First published in India by HarperVantage 2025
An imprint of HarperCollins *Publishers*
HarperCollins *Publishers* India, Cyber City, Building 10-A,
Gurugram, Haryana-122002, India
www.harpercollins.co.in

2 4 6 8 10 9 7 5 3 1

P-ISBN: 9789369891054
E-ISBN: 9789369896493

Typeset in 13/17.5 Adobe Garamond Pro
by HarperCollins *Publishers* India Pvt. Ltd

Printed and bound at
Thomson Press (India) Ltd

FSC
www.fsc.org
MIX
Paper | Supporting responsible forestry
FSC® C001695

HarperCollins *Publishers*, Macken House, 39/40 Mayor Street Upper, Dublin 1,
D01 C9W8, Ireland

To the unwavering spirit and resilience of all our liver transplant patients and their families

CONTENTS

FOREWORD

As a sportsperson we see more bad days than good. There are more sorrows than joys. And I must admit that I am a very poor loser. I used to be crestfallen after our team lost or if I failed. I encountered one such bad phase in the year 2007 when I was not picked in the World Cup squad. I was frustrated. It seemed that my world had come to an end. Such was my disappointment that a part of me was saying that I should quit cricket. I was sharing these thoughts with a childhood friend who was listening to me patiently, when he asked me to get up and come with him.

After about 20 minutes of drive, we reached a place. I had no clue where we were going. We started to walk, and I realised that it was a cremation ground, Nigambodh Ghat in Delhi. There was sorrow all around. Young and old; men and women were howling, crying as they bid final goodbyes to their deceased loved ones. I was shell shocked as I had never seen something like this. My friend told me, 'Gauti, I understand that you are disappointed for not being picked. But my friend, there is no bigger setback than death.' That incident gave me perspective.

I began to value life a lot more. I began to value my family and loved ones a lot more.

Thereafter, my respect for medical science, hospitals, doctors, nurses, caretakers and the entire medical fraternity went up a lot more. We all saw what happened during Covid. I was a member of Parliament then and saw first-hand how doctors, nurses and other members of medical fraternity worked day and night to save lives. This book is another such example where medical fraternity, the children suffering from liver diseases, and their families all teamed up to beat death. These are not only 25 stories of pediatric liver transplantation, but these are 25 sagas of hope, courage and human perseverance against all odds.

The book also illustrates how medical professionals closely witness the turbulence that patients and their families go through, becoming partners in their emotional rollercoasters. The hope of recovery, undoubtedly, is extremely mutual. The best part of this book is that like cricket, every story is real, there is no fiction, there is nothing orchestrated, nothing grey—all black and white. The authors, too, have kept everything subtle and in these times of social media hyperboles, have not glorified these tales.

Gautam Gambhir

INTRODUCTION

Advancements in medical science, on the face of it, appear to be a glorious conquest over disease and illness. The discoveries of new antibiotics to treat resistant infections, technologies to diagnose the smallest of cancers and even transplantation of organs unknown before ...

Yes, medical science does conquer. Not just disease and illness, but the immense human suffering that accompanies it, the grief that families endure and the sorrow of losing dear ones. They reflect the victory of human desire to live and of perseverance against all odds. The sacrifices that each family makes into overcoming social, economic, cultural and emotional barriers to adopt new advancements are, if not more, as significant as that of the medical fraternity in developing them.

Medical professionals closely witness the turbulence that patients and their families go through, becoming partners in their emotional roller coasters. The hope of recovery, undoubtedly, is also mutual!

It has been twenty- five years since the first successful pediatric liver transplant in India, but not many are familiar with the advances made in the field. The society at large, engrossed in the travails of its own existence, gives only a fleeting thought at new headlines about liver transplantations. This book is an effort to give the readers a peep into the lives of children transformed by pediatric liver transplantation. So immensely soul stirring have been the tales of adversity and the human resolve to get above it, the journeys of these children and their families deserve to be shared. Though each successful transplant is a hard-won battle, this book only shares the sagas of twenty-five children out of more than 500 children who have undergone a liver transplant in our program. Their lives are a reflection of how destinies can be rewritten and life triumphs over death, but not always.

THE PATHBREAKER

Dead ends force us to seek new routes. History is proof that adversity brings out the best in humanity. The potential of the human mind is beyond measure. To be a catalyst in the chemistry of breakthrough is a great honour. Just as the world celebrates Louis Brown as its first test tube baby, India boasts about its first successful pediatric liver transplant recipient in 1998, who set the stage for India to become one of the go-to countries for transplantation globally, especially South-East Asia.

Our pathbreaker was born with biliary atresia, a disease of infancy that affects about one in 15,000 babies. The biliary system is a network of ducts and channels that drains bile from the liver cells to the gall bladder. Bile is then released to the intestines. Bile helps to digest fat and carry waste products for excretion. When a baby has biliary atresia the flow of bile from the liver to the intestines is absent or blocked.

The bile gets trapped inside the liver causing damage and scarring that leads to cirrhosis. As the liver becomes scarred, it presses against the walls of the veins causing blood flow to obstruct. The result is portal hypertension (high blood pressure in the portal vein). Biliary atresia up until 1997 was a death sentence in our country and most parts of the world. Survival beyond one to two years was unfathomable. The only hope was a Kasai surgery that helps re-establish bile flow from the liver to the intestine by joining the two directly. However, it has a dismal success rate if delayed beyond two to three months of life. By the time a diagnosis was arrived at, most children would have been too old for a favourable outcome. Even with a successful surgery, the child would ultimately develop liver failure over the years in almost 70-80 per cent of the cases.

Our pathbreaker developed jaundice a few days after birth. As the jaundice increased, he underwent investigations, and a diagnosis of biliary atresia was made. He was referred for a Kasai operation and underwent the surgery at sixty-two days of life but, his liver had already been damaged. He continued to have jaundice and developed recurrent episodes of fever and abdominal distension. By eighteen months of age, he had severe growth failure and jaundice. His diseased liver failed to produce adequate protein leading to fluid build-up and severe swelling.

His only hope for survival? A new liver. His parents knew he was living on borrowed time. Their doctors had mentioned the possibility of undergoing a liver transplant abroad—an option that was way beyond their financial capacity. Luckily, a liver transplant program had recently been started at Apollo Hospital, Delhi around that time.

They overcame the financial hurdle as the hospital waived the charges, but they were still unsure. They did not want their child to die suffering in a hospital, far away from his native place and family. Should they allow him to live peacefully as long as he could? The possibility of losing the few weeks that they had was heart wrenching. Would they be able to live with that guilt?

A parent would have to undergo a major surgery to donate a liver segment as well. To subject oneself to a surgery that had never been done in India was walking down a dark, unknown path. What if they ended up losing both their son and their partner in one decision?

Liver transplant was a difficult and unsure path, nevertheless, it was the one that showed a bleak ray of promise. Hoping against hope, they clung to that miniscule ray. With tremendous courage they swallowed all their fears and chose to risk all they had to give our pathbreaker a chance. After all, great love and great achievements involve great risk.

It was a decision they celebrate to this day when their son hugs them. His mother still tears up when she recollects his post-surgery days in hospital. Our pathbreaker had a very complicated postoperative course and was in hospital for four months after his transplant. He required prolonged ventilation, developed repeated perforation of his intestines, undergoing surgery five times. He required high dose medications to treat liver rejection as his body's immune system fought the new liver. Repeated surgeries and prolonged ventilation led to infection—another challenge to overcome. But he overcame each hurdle that was thrown his way.

He survived, he thrived, he dreamt. What greater payback could it be for the medical fraternity than to have our pathbreaker come into their folds as a member, a qualified doctor? our pathbreaker chose the profession he owes his existence to. Today, at twenty-six years of age, he has completed his basic MBBS degree, is pursuing his postgraduate training and recently got married. He continues to inspire families facing the transplant option, and doctors when tough clinical scenarios daunt them. He is truly the pathbreaker.

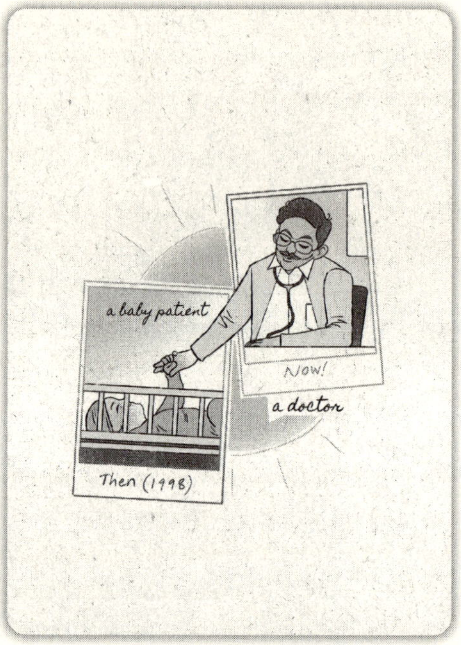

The Clinical Perspective

Our pathbreaker was the first child to undergo a living related liver transplant in India. He developed one complication after another. The transplant surgery itself had been successful with the graft and blood vessels well taken. To lose a patient to surgical issues in other organs would have been very painful. He underwent multiple other abdominal surgeries, each a potential threat to his life and our transplant program.

He has done remarkably well over the years with no late post-transplant complications. He has developed tolerance to the grafted liver and is practically off immunosuppression.

ROAD TO ADULTHOOD

Thirty-one-year-old Shoma practices accountancy away from home. He spends his weekends with his parents. He knows they cherish him and look forward to his visits. Afterall, they snatched him back from the jaws of death and nurtured him to his current blissful existence.

Shoma was just two weeks old when they noticed that he had jaundice. When it persisted longer than normal, his aunt, who was a medical student, rang the alarm bells. It's not the usual jaundice of newborns, it was something sinister. A series of tests revealed he had biliary atresia—a type where only a part of the biliary system outside the liver were present, including the gall bladder and the ducts. A variation of the classic Kasai procedure was performed using the gallbladder as a conduit to drain the intrahepatic ducts—'Gallbladder Kasai'. He was around two and a half months old at that time. Although Kasai procedure is not a permanent cure for biliary atresia, in many cases, it allows patients to grow and remain in good health for several years. This delays (or in about 25 per cent of children, eliminates) the need for a liver transplant.

Thus began Shoma and his family's battle with disease, this being first of the many hospitalizations he would endure. Post operatively, Shoma developed severe infection and was on the ventilator for a few days. After which, he remained well for about three years but then the jaundice reappeared. He was re-operated, and the classic Kasai surgery was performed. His jaundice persisted with a fluctuating course. His liver was getting progressively fibrosed and scarred, leaving him at risk for even more serious complications. He was managing with medications, but they were only supportive. He would need a liver transplant. The cost outside India was prohibitive, way beyond the reach of the family. It almost seemed they would have to watch their son die.

A report in the papers about our pathbreaker, the first successful pediatric liver transplant recipient in India in 1998, gave them hope. Shoma could be next, couldn't he? Was this the miracle they had been praying for? It sounded too good to be true, but true it was.

Shoma was six years of age when he underwent a liver transplant in 1999. He was very weak and malnourished due to his prolonged illness and was hospitalized for weeks before his transplant. The team wanted him to gain strength. He was nutritionally rehabilitated and psychologically prepared to cope with the daunting surgery.

A liver transplantation is a long abdominal surgery. The risk of intestinal perforation in view of two previous abdominal surgeries was high. He had to be operated thrice after the first week for recurrent intestinal perforation. Due to the gut leak, he had to be kept on artificial feeding through specialized preparations given intravenously. He also developed pneumonia, requiring ventilation for two weeks. His recovery consolidated the family's faith that he was divinely protected.

He walked home after four months, his medical and surgical problems sorted. But he was a changed child. Angry and aggressive after all the days in hospital, he required lots of emotional support from his family and teachers. Two years down the line, he developed tuberculosis that resulted in his brain giving him seizures. He recovered fully after regular medication. When he was eleven, their family moved to Canada, but it was his place of birth that charted his destiny. The journey was long and arduous, putting to test their physical, mental, moral and spiritual strength, but the reward made it all worth it.

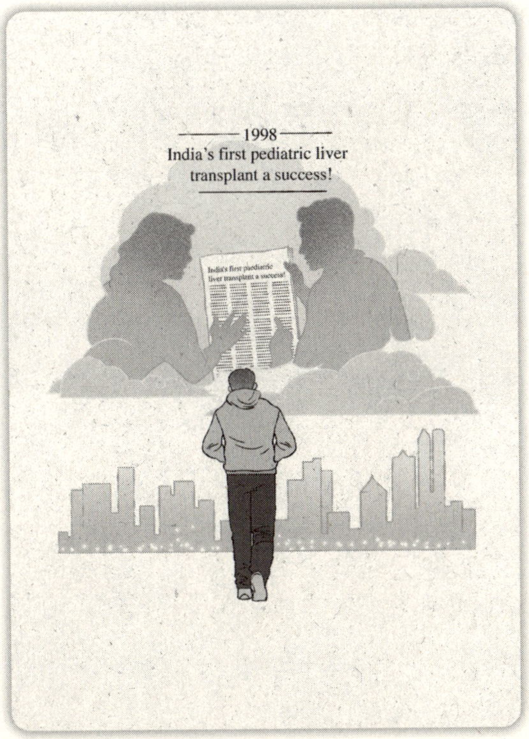

The Clinical Perspective

After our pathbreaker, Shoma proved to be our next challenge. Pre-transplant, he grew a bug in his blood and was also detected to be a silent carrier of Salmonella, the bacteria that causes typhoid. He was treated with appropriate antibiotics to eradicate the infection.

The postoperative course was tumultuous. He developed sepsis, pneumonia, gut perforations, all one after the another. He had to be kept fasting for a prolonged time to allow his gut to heal. He transiently showed features of raised intracranial pressure, raising fears of a brain haemorrhage, but thankfully, his CT head was normal.

On follow up, he had neuro-tuberculosis from which he recovered fully after adequate treatment.

THE CRICKET FAN

The list of all that is common across the Indo-Pak border is endless—genes, culture, tastes, diseases. We share the same trials and tribulations in the fields of education, economy, health and sports. We may cheer for different teams when our cricketers sweat it out in an Indo-Pak match but the love for the game is the same.

Hailing from Pakistan, Musafir Khan, loved cricket and Sachin Tendulkar as much, if not more, than any Indian. He wanted to live so that he could play cricket. The itch to watch and play cricket was stronger than the literal itch that his illness gave him. Musafir suffered from progressive familial intrahepatic cholestasis, a liver disorder that causes jaundice with severe itching and progressive liver failure.

He had suffered from intermittent jaundice since he was four months old. Like most Indians, he had been from one alternative healer to another in his quest for cure, but to no avail. By the time he turned one year old, his illness had progressed drastically causing fluid to accumulate in his abdomen. He was hospitalized and treated in Pakistan. It was only at sixteen months that he had a liver biopsy that diagnosed his illness. He was controlled on medications but over the years he had repeated episodes of jaundice, his itching became so severe he couldn't sleep or rest. Musafir was six years old when he came to India for a liver transplant with us. Little did he know that not only was he to get a liver transplant but also have an impossible dream realized.

One day he was chatting away merrily with his doctor during his assessments when he revealed his hero worship for Sachin Tendulkar. Something in his eyes struck a chord and his doctor, in addition to his transplant arrangements, went about making another set of arrangements for this young cricket enthusiast.

Sachin was in Delhi for a test match and his wife Anjali, a child specialist, was known to our fraternity. A call was made to her with a special request—a child awaiting a liver transplant worshipped Sachin, would he agree to meet him? The cricketer agreed immediately, so off went the doctors with Musafir to Sachin's hotel. Tears rolled down Musafir's eyes as he hugged his icon, took his autograph, took pictures with him and played cricket with him at the hotel for half an hour. This was the golden hour of his life, one that he would cherish all his life, if at all he lived to cherish it.

All his fears were gone. Musafir had the best wishes of his icon; he knew all would be well. And all was well indeed. Musafir had to be operated twice due to a surgical complication, he bore it bravely. He was happy when he bid adieu to India and his medical team who had given him his most treasured gifts—a new liver and memories of playing cricket with Sachin Tendulkar. He could now live blissfully; his itches had been taken care of.

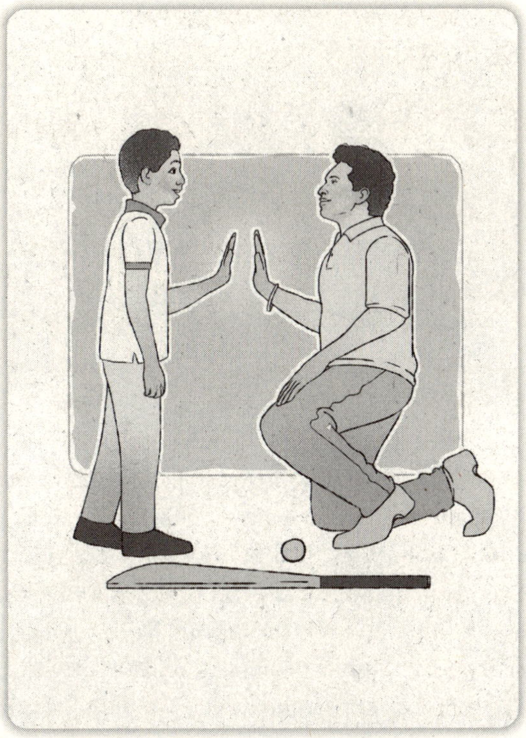

The Clinical Perspective

This disease causes severe itching that is usually refractory to medications. The impact on the child's life and psyche is tremendous. It is very gratifying to see the relief that a liver transplant brings.

TWIN BLESSINGS

Bilal Thani Ali Ahmed, a thirteen-year-old boy from Sudan, was brought to Indraprastha Apollo Hospital, Delhi with end stage renal failure. He had been passing stones in his urine since he was seven and had damaged both his kidneys requiring haemodialysis thrice a week for a year. With no urine output for twelve hours, he was in complete renal shutdown and had generalized swelling of the body due to fluid retention. He was hypertensive, his kidney tests were deranged with a serum creatinine of 5 mg/dl (normal 0.3-1.2 mg/dl) and an ultrasound of the abdomen revealed bilaterally calcified kidneys.

He was detected to have very high oxalate levels in his blood and bone marrow, leading to the diagnosis of a very rare genetic disorder, primary hyperoxaluria. This has a prevalence of only one to three per million population and results due to a biochemical defect in the liver. A deficient liver enzyme leads to excessive production of oxalate that complexes with calcium to form calcium oxalate crystals which accumulate in the kidneys, bone, heart and other organs. Earlier, a definitive diagnosis required documenting the deficient enzyme in liver tissue by obtaining a liver biopsy. But with the availability of genetic studies, we can isolate the aberrant gene by gene sequencing, thus avoiding a liver biopsy. Bilal tested positive for the AGXT gene that causes primary hyperoxaluria, thus confirming the diagnosis.

Dialysis is an inadequate treatment for these patients, as it cannot overcome the ongoing oxalate production. A kidney transplant alone doesn't suffice as the oxalates will reaccumulate and damage the new kidney as well. Cure occurs only if the deficient host liver is replaced with a liver that has the deficient enzyme, thus necessitating a combined kidney and liver transplant.

To prepare Bilal for the transplant, he was given multiple sessions of haemodialysis over a month and a half to deplete oxalate from the body. Fortunately, he did not have cardiac damage and was able to withstand the formidable surgery. His story is a glorious tale of human courage, bonds and sacrifice. His twenty-seven-year-old twin sisters were his donors, one for the kidney and another for the liver. One of the twins is a doctor and played a crucial role in mentally preparing the family for the transplant.

A team comprising of liver and renal transplant surgeons, and expert anaesthetists, performed the surgery that lasted nearly twelve hours, with the liver being transplanted first followed by the kidney. Bilal's recovery was dramatic, and he was off the ventilator within twenty-four hours. His renal parameters improved, his urine now did not show any oxalate crystals, and he was discharged within three weeks. Both his sisters also recovered well, and the jubilant family returned to their native country with a new lease of life, overwhelmed with gratitude towards our country, our doctors, modern medicine, and divine grace.

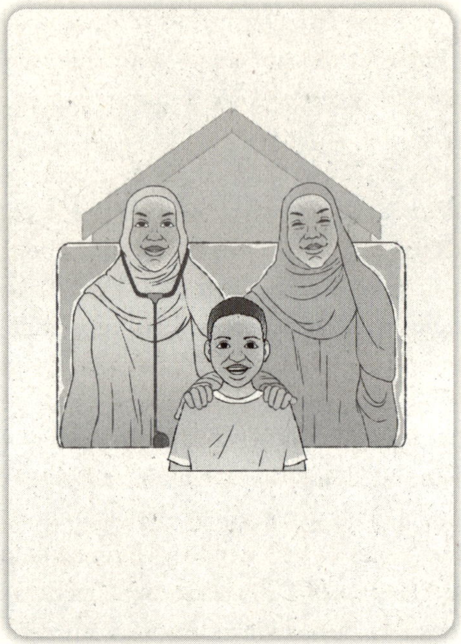

The Clinical Perspective

Arriving at a diagnosis was the first challenge. Increased oxalate excretion in the urine is the usual first line test but Bilal wasn't producing any urine at all. Oxalate crystals were detected in the eyes and genetic tests sent were confirmatory.

That he had twin sisters was a blessing. He needed two donors, one each for the liver and the kidney. It was a huge help both for the family and the transplant team that one of them was a doctor herself.

On a follow up of fourteen years, he has remained well with no significant post-transplant complications.

THE QUEST FOR DARKNESS

'Where there is despair, hope. Where there is darkness, light.' That is how the famous peace prayer by St. Francis of Assisi goes. But what if light becomes one's despair and a peaceful sleep in the dark, someone's biggest hope? How many of us take something simple like snuggling up in the sheets for a night's sleep for granted when this privilege is denied to patients with a disease called Crigler Najjar Syndrome?

This was Fatima Naji's predicament. From the moment she was born, she was to remain under direct light for hours together. This rare disease caused by an enzyme deficiency in the liver affects about one in a million population. This deficiency causes impaired excretion of a pigment called bilirubin that accumulates in the body causing severe jaundice starting within a few hours of birth. Untreated, the high bilirubin enters the brain causing fits, permanent brain damage and hearing loss. To prevent this, the jaundice needs to be controlled by keeping the baby naked, with only the eyes and genitalia covered, under lights of a specific wavelength through specially designed phototherapy machines. Phototherapy metabolizes the bilirubin allowing it to be excreted in the urine. Beyond a limit, to protect the brain, the jaundiced blood is removed from the body and simultaneously replaced with normal blood in a process called exchange transfusion.

This is the life that was given to Fatima. On the day she was born, she developed severe jaundice, and the phototherapy unit became her home. The comfort of her mother's lap was not meant for her, for she had to be under the lights, taken out only for feeding. For two months she was in hospital, undergoing repeated exchange transfusions and intensive phototherapy.

When she finally came home, she brought her phototherapy unit along with her. For sixteen to eighteen hours a day she would remain under the lights. Born in Yemen, she was the first child of a pair of young consanguineous parents, who never got a day to enjoy their parenthood. This light was their curse—one they had to learn to live with.

At around one year and six months of age, Fatima was brought to India. The only cure was a liver transplant which would be capable of producing the deficient enzyme. The parents were prepared but none of them was a suitable donor. Due to the lack of a suitable donor, they opted for a stem cell treatment instead—an experimental therapy for the disease at another city in India. Her jaundice decreased partially for a few months decreasing the need for phototherapy, but she was back to square one within six to eight months.

She was two years and three months of age when they returned to India to Apollo Hospital, Delhi. By now, she had developed some slurring of speech, difficulty in walking, and weakness in both legs indicating early brain damage. Our pediatric neurologist, an authority in her field, opined that her MRI changes could possibly reverse after a liver transplant. Any further delay and she would be a cripple forever. Her hearing was intact still.

A liver transplant for this disease had never been performed in India. Fatima's maternal aunt volunteered to donate. Fatima became the first successful liver transplant recipient for Crigler Najjar Syndrome in India. Within two weeks, her jaundice had normalized and for the first time in her twenty-seven months of living; her eyes were white instead of yellow.

About a decade and a half down the line, she is like any normal girl completing regular school, having grown beautifully into an adorable young girl, her speech and gait perfect. For years her mother's eyes would moisten when she put her to bed, kissed her goodnight and switched off the lights. She had finally been blessed with darkness.

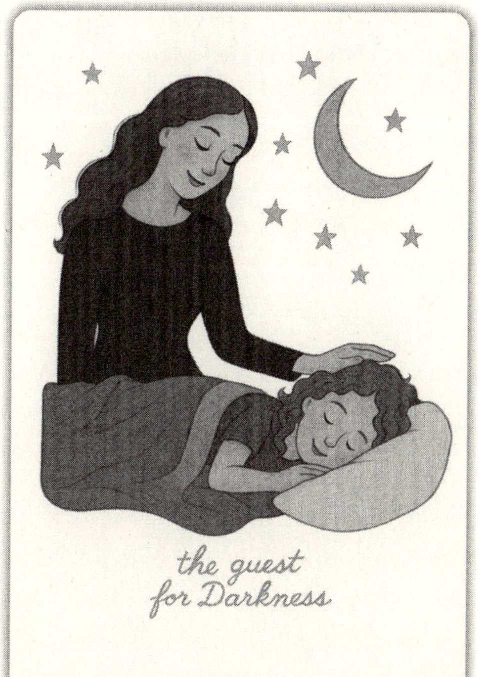

The Clinical Perspective

This was the first case of liver transplant for Crigler Najjar syndrome in our country. We were skeptical of the neurological prognosis fearing the deficits, though they were mild, would not improve. Her totally normal development and neurological recovery were well predicted by our pediatric neurologist.

Over the years, we have gone on to perform about seven transplants for this disease with excellent results. This is amongst the highest numbers for this exceedingly rare disease all over the world. However, a huge gap still exists with many continuing to be permanently crippled for want of definitive cure with a liver transplant.

THE QUIET ONE

Lord Krishna is fondly called 'Yashoda's Nanda Lal' because the mother who brought him up is revered as a greater life force than his biological mother. Amolya also had two sets of parents—the ones who gave birth to her and the ones who adopted her. She was adopted within her biological family by her parent's elder brother and wife who could not beget a child of their own. She was everyone's darling, doted on by one and all.

Just as the joy of her existence was manifold, so was the pain of seeing her suffer. Within the first year of her life, she was diagnosed with Budd Chiari Syndrome, a condition caused by occlusion of the veins of the liver. She had developed fluid collection in her abdomen and an ultrasound showed blockages in the hepatic veins. This condition leads to chronic liver disease, and she was put on regular medications. True to its nature, the disease progressed and by four years of age she had developed cirrhosis and its many complications. There was an increased pressure in the veins supplying the liver, leading to fluid accumulation in her belly, and increased risk of bleeding. She had developed hepatopulmonary syndrome (lung dysfunction secondary to liver disease, leading to shortness of breath, and breathing difficulty in upright position). She had become blue, and oxygen dependent. Liver transplantation was the only cure.

It is said that the strength of parenthood can even defeat nature. Why wouldn't her disease be defeated when she had two sets of parents ready to donate their livers for her? But here lay nature's irony. While most transplanted children receive livers from either of their parents, there was no donor for Amolya. Her biological mother was in an advanced stage of pregnancy and the other three were all rejected as donors due to medical reasons.

Her parent's cousin, a young lad who had lost his father as a child, came forward and offered to donate. His mother showed exemplary courage and magnanimity by keeping familial bonds and humanity above the maternal instinct to protect her son from any pain or risk.

Amolya's transplant went off well. For a few days, all seemed blissful till disaster struck. She had a genetic condition that gave her blood an enhanced tendency to clot, and necessitated medication to keep it thin. Its' a double-edged sword, too thin blood could cause internal bleeding. She had just received one dose but in the backdrop of intermittent blood pressure fluctuations post the surgery, she developed a massive brain haemorrhage.

Amolya was immediately operated upon and the clot in her brain removed. Gradually, she improved and the half body paralysis that had occurred showed rapid recovery. The immensely worried team began to relax as she showed progress. She became extra special, and everyone wanted to chat her up. But lo and behold, not a word was forthcoming! She would make eye contact, acknowledge with minimal gestures but was completely silent and withdrawn. Days passed; her physical recovery was almost complete. She was ready to go home but her voice was not to be heard. Her team feared she had developed aphasia which is loss of speech due to her brain injury, but the neurologist disagreed. 'The hospital environment has shut her up,' he said. After repeat CT scans of her brain proved reassuring, she was discharged.

She came to the outpatients for follow up visits, walking well, talking even better. She was the normal chatterbox her parents had known, making one demand after another, now music to their ears. She was indeed one of a kind, Amolya!

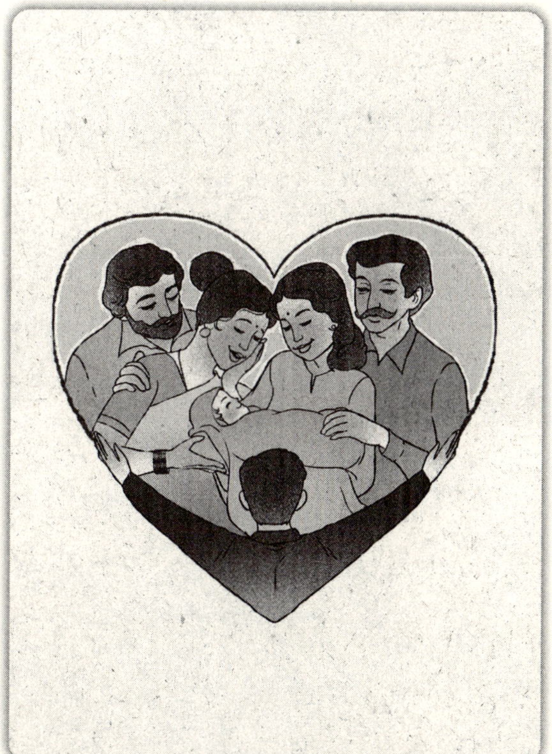

The Clinical Perspective

Brain haemorrhage is a devastating complication to have after any surgery. The liver surgery had been successful, but to send home a child cured of liver disease but paralyzed, is a predicament no team can allow. There was no plausible explanation as to what precipitated it. A single dose of antiplatelet drugs should not cause it, nor should mild intermittent hypertension. Her phase of aphasia made us feel helpless, making us wonder if we were so intimidating to the patient? Her full recovery brought immense relief.

PINK TRIUMPHS

The hospital cot was her cradle, the beeps of the monitors her rattle sounds, stethoscopes her toys, the doctors and nurses her family. For Ishani, the hospital was her home. Her parents had forgotten the joys of youth, having to grow up suddenly, sobered by the burden and enormity of Ishani's illness. Nothing could have prepared them for the suffering they would go through together.

Like all new parents, they had been overjoyed by Ishani's birth, she was God's gift to them. Full of dreams to raise her as their princess, buying her frilly frocks and fancy pink clips, they brought her home. But only if yellow could give pink a chance.

A few days after her birth, they noticed that she had yellow eyes and urine. Her stools were clay white. The possibility of a routine newborn jaundice that resolves in a few days was reassuring, but they began to worry when she was still sick well into her second month of life. Medical tests confirmed that she had biliary atresia. She needed urgent surgery and was operated at fifty-seven days of life. Thus began her war with the disease.

The cure that had been anticipated with her surgery was never to be. It only left her worse with repeated episodes of infection in her gut as it had been connected to her liver. She received multiple courses of antibiotics for the next few months. She would get a little better and be discharged from hospital, only to be back again in a week or so. This happened half a dozen times. Finally, she was then brought to Indraprastha Apollo Hospital, Delhi, emaciated and struggling for her life.

She was put on ventilatory support as her blood grew deadly bacteria for which she was treated with heavy antibiotics. Thankfully, she responded well, and her infection was controlled. But her doctors knew that her only chance for survival was to have a liver transplant. However, she weighed just 6 kg, had been ill for a long time, her liver had failed, and infection would return any time. They could not wait for her to gain weight and grow stronger for the surgery. This was the only window of opportunity. She was on top of her infection and a very high-risk liver transplant was performed.

Out went her diseased liver with all its hidden foci of infection and, along with it, her misfortune. Worst fears of her not surviving the surgery were allayed when she was wheeled out of the operation theatre after twelve daunting hours of surgery. She was a fighter, she looked better as each day passed and the real Ishani surfaced. Ishani with white eyes, soft belly with no distension, kicking her way to good health. Within three weeks she was home, never to be hospitalized again in the fifteen years that have elapsed after her transplant.

Life had triumphed, giving her the joy of childhood in her parental home, with many more to dream for. A pink graduation dress, perhaps?

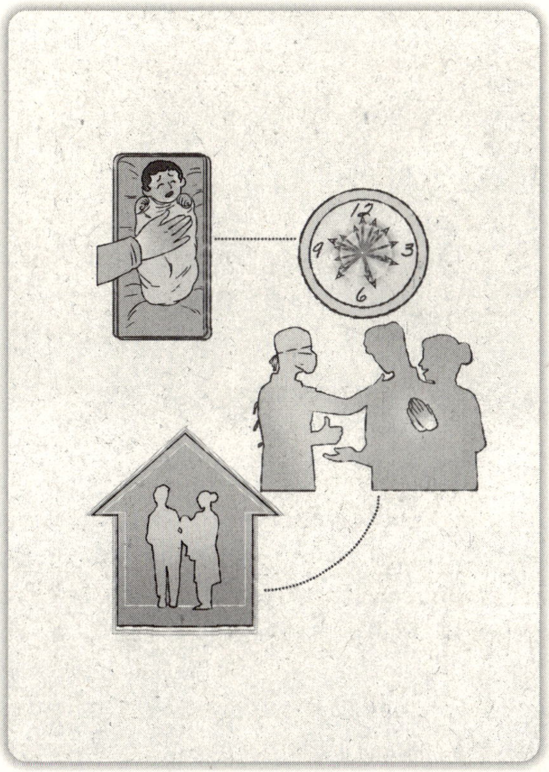

The Clinical Perspective

Ishani had been ill for too long, was very weak due to her chronic liver disease, repeated infections and prolonged hospitalization. This made her transplant very high risk and early complications like flare up of infection and vessel thrombosis were feared. However, she had a dramatic recovery after receiving the new healthy liver.

INDIAN ROOTS BECKON FROM AFRICA

'Maanvan, thandian chaavan' goes a popular Punjabi saying that describes a mother as a shade that cools and protects from the sweltering heat. Search for this solace was perhaps what brought a young Gujurati lady, hardly in her mid-twenties, to her motherland India. Her parents had migrated to South Africa before she was born but distances only make hearts grow fonder. As she landed in India, her uncles and aunts, gathered around to welcome her and her infant son, Jai.

Jai was a happy baby, his large round eyes lit up as he was showered with gifts, his 'shagun'. His mother's eyes, however, were sad as she looked at him—he was perfect, but his deep-set yellow eyes gave away his ailment.

Jai had jaundice within a few days after birth, as he suffered from biliary atresia, which then had caused his liver to fail. Why a child develops biliary atresia soon after birth, medical science has yet to fathom. All that is known is that it's universally fatal unless a partially corrective surgery is done within two months of life. The success rate of this surgery varies but liver transplant has over the last few decades revolutionized the management of this otherwise dismal disease by providing the only definitive cure. Jai's corrective surgery had failed, and his mother had come to India seeking life for her son, from the land that gave her, hers.

Her husband had stayed back to look after their other two children and her relatives from Gujarat were her only pillars of support here. She was fortunate to have a family that was so closely knit, because it was her brother-in-law who came forward to donate a part of his liver as she had been rejected as a potential donor on medical grounds.

Moving from one hospital corridor to the other, she held Jai's hand tightly as he went through the tests and assessments. Her soft voice and calm eyes spoke volumes for her inner strength as she watched her son being wheeled in for the transplant. Her usually difficult to restrain little one was engulfed in tubing, deep asleep under the effect of anaesthesia, when he returned after the ten-hour surgery. But he would soon return to his naughty self as his anaesthesia effect wore off. He was off the ventilator within a few hours, smiling reassuringly at his mother. It was as if he could sense the turmoil in her heart that she concealed from the outer world.

Like mother, like son. Jai was a brave little lad and would cry briefly when pricked for blood samples and then return to his calm demeanor. Only hunger would unsettle him, and he was cheerful once feeds were started three days after the surgery. He became a darling of the nurses who wouldn't tire of playing with him.

The gods favour the humble and Jai recovered well. He was discharged in three weeks, his eyes perfectly pearly white, carrying only the surgical scar on his tummy as a memento of the terrible illness he was born with and had conquered in his native land.

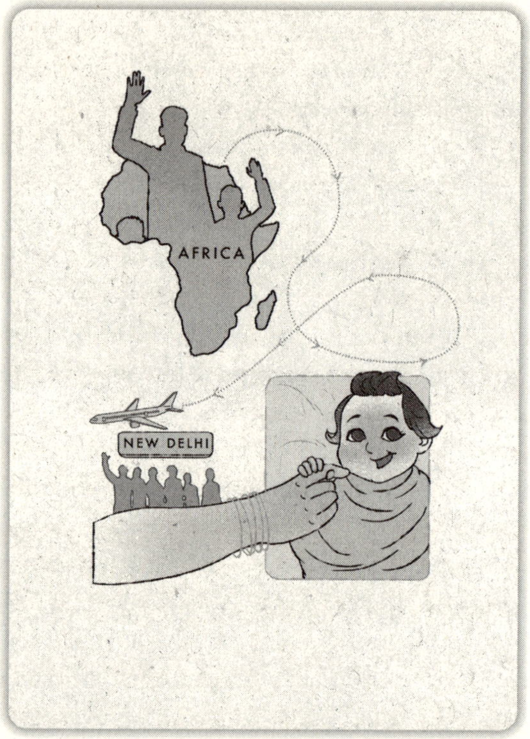

The Clinical Perspective

Jai, thankfully, did not develop any major complications. He had intermittently high potassium levels for which he required a potassium binder. Jai easily drank the medication mixed with his feeds and was an exceptionally co-operative and an easy to manage baby.

THE CAMBODIAN CHAMP AND HIS CHEERLEADER

'Doctor! doctor! Look! Borai is dancing! He is hiding and peeping from behind the curtains! Look at him!' The nurse beamed with joy as she ran through the ward corridor to share the news. The doctor was quick to capture the moment in his mobile and the mother was in tears, this time, of happiness.

Countless tears had been shed on countless occasions while struggling to save her only living child. Four miscarriages, a child lost in infancy to an undiagnosed illness, a broken marriage, all alone in a foreign land with a child ill from birth—the strongest of humans would have broken in such a predicament, but not Borai's mother. One of the biggest joys in life is to love and be loved. Borai was the one to love her back and she would do all in her power to have him live.

She first come to India from Cambodia when Borai was about a year and a half. He had biliary atresia and had a corrective surgery at two months of age in Singapore, but his liver functions continued to deteriorate. He had repeated episodes of jaundice with fever and when he began to vomit blood, he was advised for an urgent liver transplant. Fortunately, funds were not an issue. The family chose to come to Delhi.

Borai underwent a liver transplant and was discharged within three weeks. His liver functions improved rapidly, and we sent home this little bundle of joy, his eyes sparkling with the hint of mischief, his laughter so infectious that the hospital gloom would be uplifted within seconds of being with him.

But the troubles he was born with didn't go away with his liver. After remaining well for about twenty months, Borai developed swelling all over his body and was detected to have kidney dysfunction. He was back with us; his blood pressure was high, and his normally cheery nature was drowned in his restlessness.

Anxiety was writ large on the faces of the transplant team. Their worst fears were confirmed with the medical and kidney biopsy reports. Borai had developed chronic renal disease due to transplant associated thrombotic microangiopathy, a condition where the small blood vessels get occluded due to damage to their inner lining. This is a very rare but devastating complication of transplantation with mortality ranging from 60-90 per cent.

Medications were changed, treatments instituted but to no avail. Borai's kidney function continued to deteriorate and soon he was on haemodialysis with no option but to undergo a renal transplant. One of his maternal uncles came forward to donate his kidney and the mother steeled herself to consent for his high-risk surgery that fortunately, went off well. But Borai's troubles were far from over. He continued to have renal dysfunction and had multiple sessions of plasma exchange, intravenous steroids, and high-end novel therapies were instituted to save the new kidney. He picked up a urine infection, developed spiking high fevers requiring prolonged antibiotics. He was in the intensive care unit on his birthday, had fever when he cut the cake, yet was happy playing with the toy car his doctors had bought him. The injections, the monitors, the nurses had somehow integrated into his life and the pain couldn't subdue his joyous spirit. That was what triumphed ultimately when his new kidney started working well, his complications controlled, he danced in his room, his pranks were back and so was the long-lost smile on his mother's face. He had won, a mother's resilience had paid off and he went home after a four-month long hospital stay, all hale and hearty.

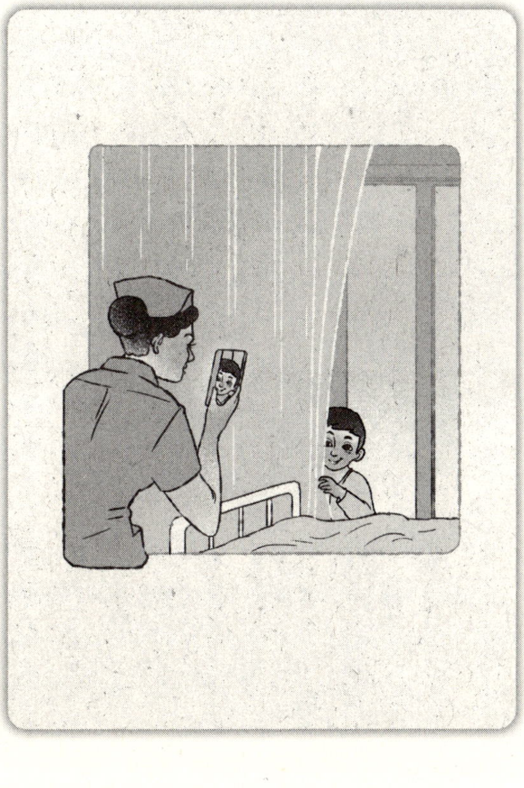

The Clinical Perspective

Thrombotic microangiopathy has been reported frequently after stem cell and bone marrow transplants but is exceedingly rare after liver transplantation. After one organ transplant, he needed another—a nightmare for any family and treating unit. He needed strategizing on multiple therapies to control the angiopathy and make the kidney transplant feasible and successful whilst also protecting the grafted liver. The situation was very challenging, and we really feared losing Borai.

FATHER-SON: EACH OTHER'S SAVIOURS

The doctor's measuring tape doubled up as a tailor's tape for taking measurements for Vivek's clothes. He was being discharged and his doctors, along with giving him a new liver, wanted to dress him up in new clothes. 'Please don't bring anything in red,' he whispered in his mother's ear to convey to his doctor, who was now off from the ward round to proceed for the mall round shopping for Vivek.

Some people evoke sympathy, others evoke empathy. Vivek was one who evoked pure love and deep affection. He was too blessed to be sympathized with. Despite his illness, there was never a moment where you could catch him awake without a smile on his face. Ever radiant, ever beaming, ever content, the gleam in his eyes never gave away his tale of suffering.

Aged eleven years, he had been in and out of hospitals multiple times over the last four years. The first episode had occurred when he was barely three years of age, but they had progressively grown worse as he'd grown older. Repeated episodes of fever, jaundice, abdominal pain and vomiting brought him from a small village near Jalandhar to Ludhiana and then to the Post Graduate Institute of Medical Education and Research (PGIMER), Chandigarh in his quest for a cure. A diagnosis of primary sclerosing cholangitis was arrived at, a condition in which the draining channels for bile become beaded and narrowed, leading to bile accumulation in the liver and subsequent tissue damage. With the non-complaining temperament that he had; Vivek patiently endured seven endoscopic attempts by his doctors to put in a stent across his main blockage. As a last resort, an external diversion was created that drained his bile into a bag, attached with a tubing, to his gall bladder.

To live with a bag attached, liver already damaged and shrunken, no school, no play—was this to be Vivek's fate? He deserved better and the universe ensured he got his due.

He needed a liver transplant, that was his only chance of a life worth living. An alcoholic out-of-work father, two elder school-going sisters, a mother who supported the family with her peon's salary barely making ends meet. Where were the means to save Vivek?

His doctors needn't have despaired. The entire universe had conspired to help Vivek. The liver transplant team at Indraprastha Apollo Hospital offered a free transplant, in which the bed charges and fees would be waived off, with the patient needing to pay only for medicines and consumables. That would cut the cost to about half (Rs 6,00,000), but that too was beyond their means. In true community spirit, his village and the panchayat took on the challenge to raise money. A public appeal was issued, several rounds of kabaddi matches were organized to raise funds and sanctions were obtained from the Punjab Chief

Minister's relief fund. Rs 1,00,000 each was donated by kind parents of two other patients. Soon the required sum was in the kitty.

With the funds arranged, evaluation of the mother as a donor was started. After all the positivity, no one was prepared for this setback—even though she had no symptoms, her main vessel supplying the liver was found to be blocked, making her unfit to donate. Both the sisters were still minors. Tears rolled down her eyes as she foresaw all her efforts go down the drain.

Little did she realize, God had grander plans for her. A new life awaited not only her son but also her husband, whom this challenge reformed completely. To be able to donate a part of his liver, he would have to abstain from alcohol for at least three months. Post donor surgery, if that happened, alcohol would be taboo, as it would harm his regenerating liver. Love for his son proved stronger than his love for alcohol. What years of coercing and pleading by his family could not achieve, the desire to see his son live, did. Not a drop of alcohol went down his throat in the next three months and he was then cleared as a donor by his surgeons.

What could go wrong with Vivek after having surmounted odds of such gravity? All went well, he went home looking dapper in his new clothes.

He has now graduated in hotel management and recently emigrated to Canada, his father—now a teetotaler—earns reasonably as a carpenter, his mother and sisters have never been happier, and the village panchayat never felt prouder. From the greatest adversities emerge the greatest success stories, such are life's ways!

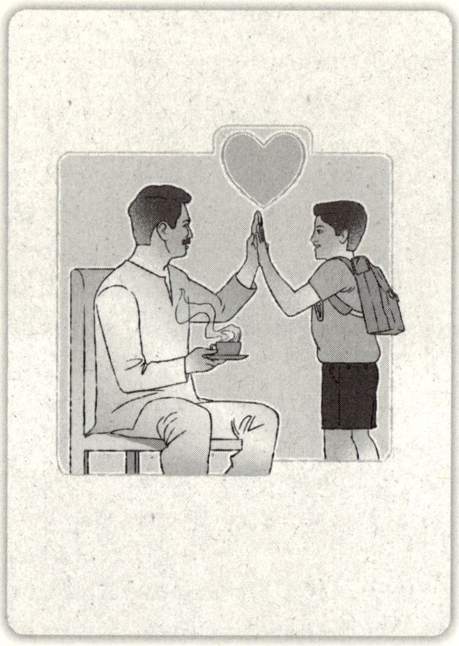

Clinical perspective:

Vivek and his family had suffered for almost eight years due to his illness. Recurring at progressively decreasing intervals ever since he was three, for the last four years he had been ill every two to three months. By the time he was diagnosed, he already had portal hypertension. As stenting had failed despite repeated attempts, a cholecystostomy had been done that was an open channel for infection and tended to block.

Vinay's liver transplant was a success—medically and socially. He became a model for other patients from the poor strata of society, bridging them from despair to hope.

'AYUBOWAN'

'Ayubowan'—May you have the gift of long life! With this traditional Sri Lankan greeting, Dhanush was welcomed to his place of birth by his grandparents. Just as this tear shaped island country is the sparkling jewel of the Indian Ocean, so was Dhanush, the jewel of his family, doted by one and all.

His parents had migrated to UAE, and it was his skin condition that had brought them on this trip back home. Dhanush suffered from vitiligo, a skin disease that causes white patches on the body. With faith on their country's traditional heritage, they banked on an alternative medicine therapist to try and heal him with herbal medication. Sadly, it became the source of their nightmare.

He had been on his herbal medications for a few weeks when he began to have fever followed by vomiting and jaundice. He had developed hepatitis, i.e., inflammation of the liver. His parents took him back to Abu Dhabi for medical care but his condition progressively deteriorated. He had developed acute liver failure and was susceptible to life threatening bleeding or coma, if his liver function continued to deteriorate any further. He needed an urgent liver transplant.

Emergency contact with the team of liver specialists at Indraprastha Apollo Hospitals was made, and he was flown to India. It was inferred from his clinical course and diagnostic workup that he had developed liver failure due to the herbal medications; all tests for an infective cause or underlying silent chronic liver disease were negative.

Preparations were started and he was admitted to the intensive care unit. It was a herculean task to care for him. He would speak little and would resist blood tests with all his might. His long dark curly hair made the staff mistake him time and again for a girl, causing him to sulk further. Only his mother could understand his agitated state of mind behind his quiet persona. She was his magic charm and became his donor, giving him life twice.

The transplant surgery was a success, and he was off the ventilator within a few days. When all seemed fine, arose another problem. He would not accept his oral medicines. He hated them. According to his mother, he had always been averse to taking medicines. He would just shut his mouth and require coercing for hours together, becoming agitated when forced. After undergoing a transplant, one needs to take regular medications, to prevent the body from rejecting the new liver. For a few days, his oral feeding tube was not removed after surgery so that he could be given his medications. The magic charm that his mother was, she gradually and lovingly brought him around, and he slowly overcame his strong aversion to medicines.

By the time of discharge, his syrups didn't anger him, the needles and syringes didn't terrify him. All he wanted was to go home to live the life he had been blessed with.

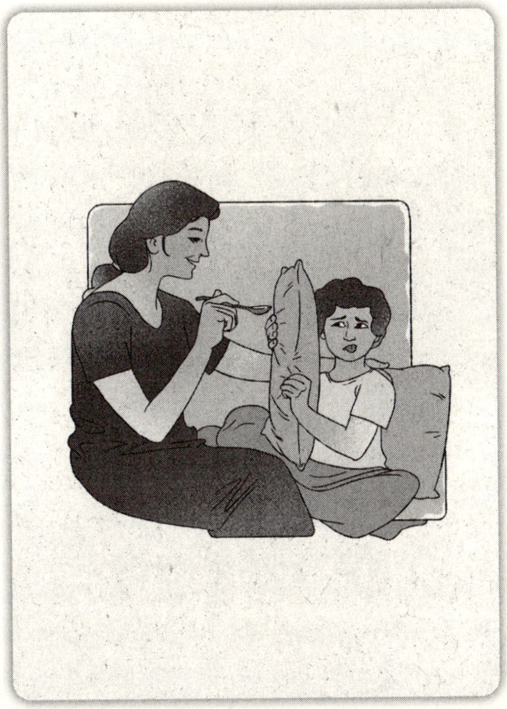

The Clinical Perspective

Acute liver failure is a grave medical emergency as the mortality risk is very high. An urgent liver transplant must be arranged before the patient develops complications involving the brain, kidneys and other organs that would render a transplant unfeasible and/or futile. Dhanush had to be airlifted to our hospital from UAE at a very short notice. Meticulous preparations ensured he underwent a timely transplant.

GOD'S GIFT

Imprisonment sentences for the severest crimes end in ten to fourteen years. Simran's mother often wondered what she had done to deserve a banishment from motherhood. She had been married for almost seventeen years and was yet to beget a child of her own. It is said that motherhood completes a woman and brings out the best in her. She had suffered repeated miscarriages that had completely drained her body and soul. Pregnant again, she prayed fervently for the successful outcome of this pregnancy. But she had been praying for years and years, she had begun to ask herself—was there a God?

The cry of her newborn baby seemed like a call from the heavens above to uphold her faith. She had never been happier! No sound sweeter! Her husband wept like a baby. They had finally become proud parents to their newborn jewel, a baby girl, Simran.

Sadly, their joy was short-lived. They had not even settled into their newfound roles, or learnt how to change the diapers properly before their visits to the hospitals began again. Simran had jaundice. At five months of age, she vomited blood and was hospitalized in Islamabad. She was detected to have progressive familial intrahepatic cholestasis, a condition in which liver cells are less able to secrete a digestive fluid called bile. Buildup of bile in the liver cells leads to liver failure.

She would require regular medications, but there was no way to prevent her liver disease from progressing. She had developed portal hypertension and had repeated episodes of bleeding from her gut necessitating blood transfusions and endoscopies. Every bleeding episode was a potential threat to her life.

Her parents were devastated. It seemed like a sword always dangled over their head. Her mother would go paranoid in fear. She was all but three years in age, what years of prayers had brought seemed to be slipping out of her hands. Questions plagued her mind, had she asked for something that was not meant for her? Was the joy of motherhood not destined for her? Is that why they were suffering? Could God be so ruthless? She would go crazy with grief. Was a gift, a gift at all if it was to be snatched away so soon?

But Simran was destiny's child. She was meant to live. Her doctors in Pakistan advised her for a liver transplant. It was her only hope. Her parents were terrified of such a major high-risk surgery. They chose to put their trust in the Divine and came to India for a liver transplant.

The surgery was a success, and she recovered wonderfully. She did have postoperative infections that were treated well. She went home after about five weeks in hospital. Finally, life for Simran and her parents had begun.

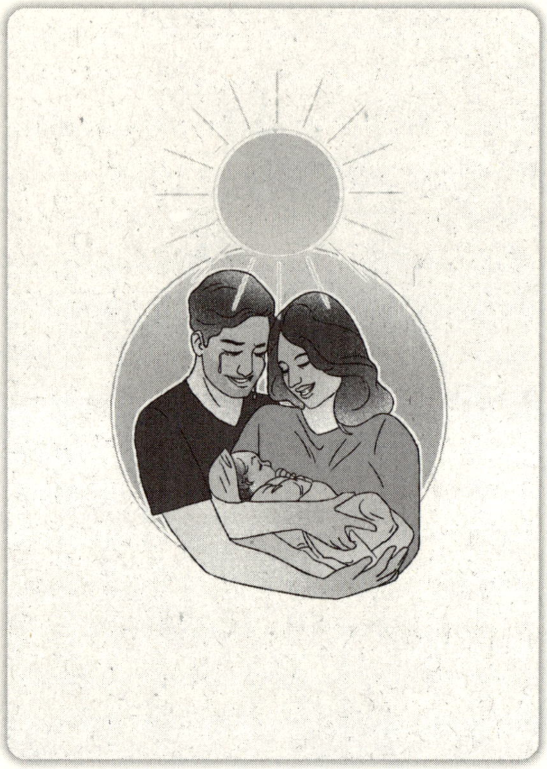

The Clinical Perspective

Post-transplant Simran developed chickenpox. She did receive prophylaxis but still suffered the infection. As all post-transplant patients are on medications to suppress their immunity and chickenpox is highly contagious, an outbreak in the postsurgical unit would have been devastating. She was immediately isolated, and all precautions taken.

THE MIRACLE KID

Enrapturing victory, success and joy, his name 'Praful' embodies all that he stands for. His journey is a miracle that truly enraptures our heart and soul, leaving even the hardest non-believers faithful with a belief that there stands a power far greater than you and I.

Second year into their marriage, Praful's parents were worried. They were hoping for a baby. The elders in the family, like most ones in Indian families, had started enquiring for the 'good news'. A series of tests and visits to the gynecologist shattered their dreams. Praful's mom, Navita, had severe tubal blocks in both tubes, surgical correction was tried but they were told a spontaneous conception would be 'impossible'. A natural pregnancy without assisted reproduction techniques would be a 'miracle'.

We have all heard fairytales and fables about miracles. Do they really happen? Aren't they just figments of imagination handed down generations to reinforce a belief in a higher force? In Navita's case, there were miracles, not one but one after another, that unfolded in her life. The first was Praful's natural conception.

Navita's happiness knew no bounds when she realized she was expecting her first baby, the 'impossible' had happened. Praful came into this world bringing joy and ecstasy into their dejected hearts. A few weeks of blissful parenting before their joys were replaced by fears. Soon after birth, Praful developed jaundice that refused to go away. Detailed evaluations in the third month of his life revealed he had biliary atresia wherein the biliary system, a network of channels that drains bile produced in the liver to the gall bladder has blockages causing liver damage due to bile stasis.

Over the next few months, he developed progressive liver failure and was practically in and out of hospital. They were referred for a liver transplant, without one he didn't stand a chance. His parents were devastated. They had thanked their stars for his birth, wondered what past good deeds had manifested this miracle into their lives. Was their faith in the Divine being tested? They couldn't afford a liver transplant; they couldn't afford to lose Praful either. Praful was too precious to be lost, their hearts bled at their predicament.

Praful was too precious to this universe as well. Another miracle was about to unfold, a person unknown and unrelated to them was about to become his guardian angel. The transplant team had put in an appeal on national television seeking financial help. Herein, stepped in a person with a heart of gold, one who is revered by his fans for his cricketing skills, his wit and his down to earth persona. The prominent media personality put in Rs 18,00,000 to cover for his surgery and the recurring lifetime cost of his medications without letting out a word for publicity. To give is great, to give silently is divine. The only bank that can never go bankrupt is the bank of selfless love.

The hospital chose not to charge for the transplant apart from the Rs 6,00,000 to be spent on the consumables. The remaining twelve would be put into a fixed deposit and the interest pay for the monthly immunosuppression medications. Does this bring us to the end of the story? All hurdles sorted, successful surgery and happily ever after? Man proposes, God disposes. There was another miracle waiting to happen, one that would jeopardize all their plans, that seemed more of a setback than a blessing.

All pretransplant assessments for Praful were complete. Navita, being the same blood group as him was to be the liver donor. Her ultrasound abdomen was done as a part of assessment before surgery, but it left her flabbergasted. She was in the third month of another pregnancy, one that she was totally unaware of. She had been declared infertile at one point of time, and here she was with another pregnancy!

She wept her heart out and steeled herself. She had to save Praful, and she contemplated an abortion. She asked to confirm how soon after an abortion could she go in for the donor surgery. Today, she credits the life of both her children to our team. We put our foot down, no abortion. She would not be the donor. There was no guarantee Praful would survive the liver transplant, was she prepared to live with the loss of both her children if Praful didn't make it?

As if the whole Universe had conspired to bless them with a happy family, Praful had another guardian angel up his little sleeve. An aunt with Praful's blood group showed great magnanimity and came forward to donate a part of her liver. After all these miracles, how could the miracle surgery that has revolutionized the course of this disease ever go wrong? Both Praful and his aunt recovered very well after their surgeries.

More than a decade and a half after Praful's transplant, with his younger brother in tow, they constitute of one blissful family. They have been truly blessed beyond their fondest dreams. They live in gratitude for Providence has brought them their highest good, for their greatest joy.

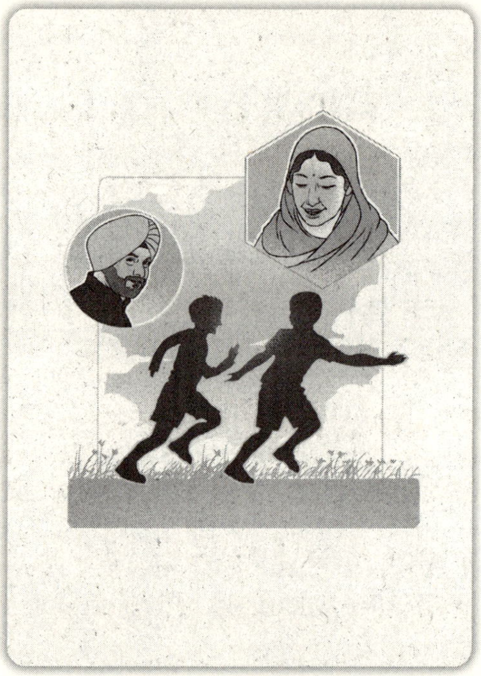

Clinical perspective

Praful has had a miracle run in the clinical context as well. He had a smooth surgery and postoperative course. On follow ups, he has done remarkably well with no late post-transplant complications.

THE GOLDEN SALMAN

Azaan Ahmed was eleven years old when he walked in with his mother into the transplant outpatient services. 'His friends call him the golden boy or the sunflower boy because of his colour' was how his mother introduced her smiling, handsome, plump, yellow son. An articulate and educated lady, she narrated the tale of their journey spanning eleven years in a very composed and dignified manner.

'This is a journey we didn't opt for, wish for, or aim for'. No parent would choose to be in their predicament, to have an all-healthy child with a well-functioning liver but deeply jaundiced within hours of birth due to an inborn enzyme deficiency. Patients born with Crigler Najjar disease suffer with severe jaundice that can potentially irreversibly damage the brain due to pigment deposition when the levels exceed defined limits. Phototherapy, that provides special lights at a certain wavelength to decrease the levels, becomes the lifesaving lifelong companion.

Azaan remained jaundiced for all these eleven years, every single day of his life. Apart from his golden yellow colour, he was like any other child. This colour kept him naked for ten to twelve hours every day. He would be in the sun every morning and evening while attending school in between, every night he slept naked under the home phototherapy machine. Ensuring adequate phototherapy while continuing education, exercise, partying, being amongst friends, neighbours and relatives is no mean task. Yet so meticulous was his care that his jaundice remained controlled adequately enough for him to suffer no neurological injury.

'Salman Khan, put on your shirt' teased his friends, collating him to the quintessential Bollywood hero popular for baring his torso. As he grew older, his parents were increasingly worried. Managing phototherapy lights that could provide the requirements of a boy his size was getting progressively difficult. He would soon step into adolescence; how would he take his illness at this most fragile stage of life? A liver transplant, by providing a liver capable of producing the deficient enzyme, could be his only permanent cure. Neither of the parents could be his liver donors. Strict physical fitness requirements of his father's profession as a defense personnel, and medical constraints with his mom, made them live with a feeling of desperation and helplessness.

Years had passed waiting and struggling when a breakthrough came with his maternal uncle voluntarily coming forward to donate. His mother planned her travel to India from Pakistan, with her brother and son, who would both undergo major surgeries. She needed her husband by her side at this most testing time. Her apprehensions were set aside when seeing their plight, a visa was readily issued by the Indian authorities to a Pakistan Air Force officer.

Azaan recovered very well post-transplant as his jaundice rapidly cleared. From the golden boy emerged a fair handsome young lad with blushing cheeks. His jaundice was gone but he held on to his Salman connection. He had been called the 'Shirtless Salman Khan' all his life, after all. He was in India, and he now wanted to see him in person. He wished to travel to Mumbai and see him shoot on the sets. 'We have a visa only for Delhi, and also you can't be in crowded places so soon after surgery,' reasoned his mother. Mentioned as a joke during the rounds, this became a non-medical priority for his medical team to address.

Azaan's journey was a remarkable one. A one in a million disease, exemplarily well managed for more than a decade, now cured in his mother's words due to a 'humanitarian effort that crossed the border, uniforms, services, enmity, and religions for the promotion of dignity of humankind'. Did it not merit a special meeting from Salman Khan himself? It definitely did, and the 'Being Human' ambassador promptly agreed to meet him. Special short visas for a trip to Mumbai were arranged. Azaan ecstatically met his star who spent an hour with him making him feel like a hero. He indeed was one in his own right. Just like the role of a wrestler Salman personified in the film 'Sultan', Azaan too had wrestled (albeit with a rare disease) and won out of sheer grit and self-belief.

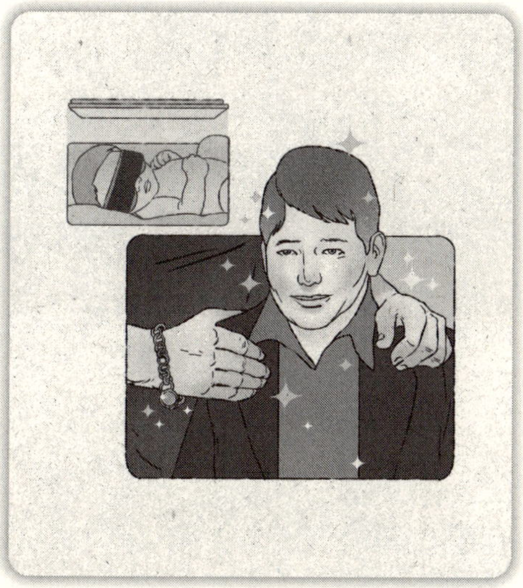

Clinical perspective:

Azaan had been very well managed for his disease despite the practical difficulties of phototherapy in a growing child. His jaundice had been controlled to safe limits and he had no neurological complications, thanks to the exemplary discipline and dedication of the family. The transplant surgery went through without any major complications and his jaundice rapidly cleared. He remains well on follow up with greatly improved quality of life due to freedom from his constant phototherapy.

THE DEMONS ARE BACK

'Doctor Sahib, how can I eat food that I don't like? Please explain to my mumma,' said Paul in his usual nonchalant and authoritative manner. Hospital food refusal was his chief complaint on every medical round, the first few minutes would always be about his meals. He had to have chicken and mutton delicacies of his taste, specially prepared for him by the hospital chef or his mother. His demands were readily and happily complied with, a pleasure to fulfil for a child who had overcome imminent death and was fighting stage IV liver cancer.

Paul, a resident of Pakistan, aged six years, a student of class 1 was the darling of his family. Intelligent and quick witted above his years, he was doted on by one and all in the family and his neighbourhood. A seemingly trivial tummy ache could not hold him back from his school or his games. As the pain persisted, his dad, who is a radiology technician himself, took him to hospital for an ultrasound abdomen. Misfortune's silent approach was soon to be demonstrated. Paul's well and healthy demeanor masked the vulnerabilities of human existence, the fragility of our happiness, the deceptiveness of fate; this happy soul carried a large tumour in his liver, a time bomb ticking away silently in his belly.

His distraught parents, a lovely young couple, prepared themselves for the emotionally, physically, financially and spiritually draining journey ahead. A biopsy was scheduled to secure the diagnosis and chart a treatment plan. Paul had a massive bleed from the tumour after biopsy, he bled into his abdomen and lungs. His parents and doctors were devastated, death seemed to have come knocking before offering him a chance to therapy. His devout parents prayed fervently, calling out to his saviour, his Good Shepherd for his redemption. A chest tube was put in to decompress the lungs. Emergent embolization procedure succeeded in blocking the bleeding vessel thus halting the march of death. Paul had won his first battle.

The tussle with his disease would now play out at another level, in another country, that was once one with theirs, where common cultural threads would welcome him in as its own. Paul took to India as fish to water as he stormed into the hearts of the medical staff. His CT scans and biopsy had confirmed the diagnosis of stage IV hepatoblastoma that would require chemotherapy and a subsequent liver transplant due to multisegment involvement. However, he was in a very critical state with right side pneumonia, fluid in the space around his lungs, a massive collection of clotted blood in his liver besides the tumour. A chest tube was put in again and he required potent intravenous antibiotics. He remained in hospital for about a month and was started on chemotherapy once infection was controlled and the chest tube removed.

Paul received multiple cycles of chemotherapy to shrink his tumour. He would be in hospital for two days every two weeks, breezing in with him an air of infectious laughter, happiness and therapeutic positivity for all around. The healing energy he radiated as he healed physically seemed saintly. Despite full insight into his illness at this tender age, he was never dejected or depressed.

With his tumour well shrunken after chemotherapy and no evidence of any spread beyond the liver on his whole-body scan, a liver transplant would be the final curative step. His transplant went off as well as he had taken his illness. Paul was discharged within twenty days with no evidence of any residual tumour burden. The family had spent almost six months in India, having celebrated Christmas and New Year here. Easter was celebrated in hospital while recuperating post-transplant. Himself feeling resurrected, Paul went back home with memories of the taste of Karim's, the architectural beauty of the Red Fort and Jama Masjid, with three bags full of new clothes and a 28 kg bag of toys, apart from the two segments of liver that his mother had gifted him.

'Hope is the physician of every misery,' goes an Irish proverb. 'The human spirit is stronger than anything that can happen to it,' said CC Scott. Beautiful words that give great courage. But what do you say if you have put in all the fight, won the battle, celebrated the victory but are struck again? Struck again by the demons you thought you had fought away, the demons that lay deceptively dormant, only to stealthily creep back into the existence you were just beginning to gather back?

Barely two months after his transplant, Paul developed severe back pain and was detected to have three of his back bones crumbling due to recurrence of his tumour, a large mass in his spine pressing the nerves causing paralysis of his legs. Why the best people often have terrible lives is beyond comprehension. Paul, the most endearing and adorable kid, one never to be put down now lay in excruciating pain. On medications for pain control, on salvage chemotherapy and radiotherapy, fighting again, praying for a miracle to manifest for cure, it was heart wrenching to walk with him in his suffering.

Greatly humbling the medical fraternity, Paul's poignant state and ultimate death represent that there are miles to go for medical therapies despite all the advances and victories. Words cannot define the emotional and psychological turmoil that medical personnel bravely endure in their daily tug of war with death.

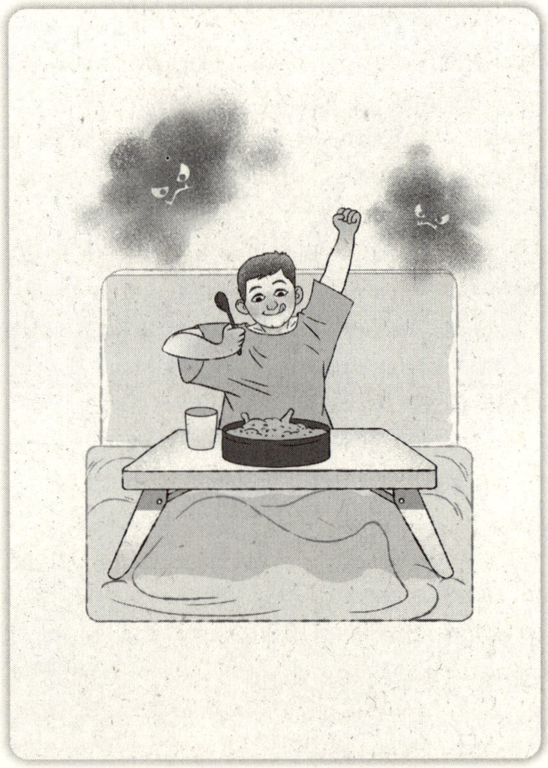

The Clinical Perspective

Paul was a medical challenge as he was admitted in a very fragile state. He already had infected lungs and the clotted blood in his liver would be a very potent medium for bacteria to grow. Trying to drain it would be very hazardous, entailing a high risk of torrential life-threatening bleed akin to the one previously experienced. Paul responded very well to therapy and the sepsis was controlled. The tumour was very chemo-sensitive and shrunk rapidly. Being multifocal, liver resection was not an option, and he was transplanted after minimizing the tumour burden and ruling out other organ involvement. He was thoroughly evaluated with a whole-body PET scan to rule out tumour activity beyond the liver. The recovery was remarkable with no major complications. Postoperatively, his serum AFP, a tumour marker for hepatoblastoma rapidly normalized indicating tumour eradication. The liver remained tumour free with no local recurrence. The recurrence at a new site due to micrometastasis that escaped detection was medically devastating and deeply demoralizing. Chances for cure after such a recurrence are dismal and we are left in the painful predicament of a healthy disease-free liver in a body ravaged by tumour recurrence.

THE IMPOSSIBLE ONE

'Oh my God! Are you really going to take up this baby for liver transplant?' exclaimed our pediatric hematologist in a horrified manner. Her patient was admitted on the other bed in the twin sharing room where baby Vae (fondly called VC) was being optimized and evaluated for a liver transplant. Deeply jaundiced, all skin and bones, with a hugely bloated belly due to fluid accumulation in her abdomen, a complication of chronic liver failure. She weighed barely 3.5 kg at nine months, inclusive of the weight of her abdominal fluid. Her parents are closely associated with a church in the Philippines where VC's dad is a lay minister assisting with the mass every Sunday. A simple, devout happy couple, they joyously welcomed their third daughter. As is usual in such cases, the early signs of a liver problem were missed and the jaundice that was noted in the second month was evaluated only by the time she was four months of age. Her liver biopsy was suggestive of biliary atresia with early signs of liver cirrhosis. The family was told that a few months down the line she would need a liver transplant that was not available for children in their country. They would need to travel to Taiwan that would cost around a 100,000 USD, an amount they wouldn't be able to raise in the few months that she had. In her father's words: 'We were so disheartened that day, as if the world toppled on us. We don't know where we could get that large amount of money to save our child's life, I had a stable job, but it would be impossible to raise that amount for a year or two. I was thinking then to give-up our child, we could not bear how she is suffering from her ailment. I was angry with God, I questioned Him why he let these things happen to us. But then I talked to Him, and offered everything to him, asking him to help us save our child's life. Suddenly I had a clear mind and heart, as if I heard him saying I will take care of you and your child. Trust me!'

A few patients had recently travelled to our hospital for a liver transplant from their country. VC's parents happened to bump into one of them in their hospital as they shared the specialist's contact who cared for them. The initial experience in India for the few who had been transplanted was very good, with the cost being just about a third of that in Taiwan where most previous transplants were being referred to. Her parents believed that this was the answer their prayers and faith had brought, and India became their hope, they set on to raise the target amount. They sold different items like t-shirts, bear towels, candles, crinkles and others. They also organized movie screenings, golf tournaments and gave out a lot of solicitation letters. Help was forthcoming from their relatives, friends, officemates and their catholic community. The community came together remarkably to help them every step of the way—fund raising, making travel and stay arrangements, providing contingency support, getting grants. Even their air tickets were sponsored by the Senator. Another donor provided them monetary assistance that helped complete their needed funds and gave them an extra budget, which was later used to buy a one year supply of baby VC's medicine.

Our surgeon had visited their country and made the special effort to visit VC in the hospital, where she was admitted to drain the fluid from her belly. The doctors there were skeptical about her transplant due to her severely malnourished state and advanced liver failure. However, taking up the challenge, and risking loss of faith in his abilities in the event of an adverse outcome, in a community that was still testing its waters in our transplant program, he selflessly chose to take up her case and advised to expedite her transfer to India.

We put in a nasogastric tube from her nostril into her tummy to give her calorie dense feeds, but the weight gain was not as desired. Her evaluations revealed she suffered from cystic form of biliary atresia, where huge cysts had developed inside the liver. A few of them could be seen and felt as lumps over her abdomen. As there is high risk of cyst infection or rupture, it was decided to take her up for transplant, though she was just about 4.6 kg, despite the aggressive nutritional rehabilitation instituted. The portal vein that supplies blood to the liver was also very narrow and thrombosed; this was considered a contraindication to transplant till recently. Newer advancements in surgical techniques, including some innovations of our surgeons, had enabled them to successfully transplant babies' recipients with very narrow or blocked portal veins. The confidence of the surgical team helped boost the courage of her parents, who accepted all the risks having surrendered the outcome to Divine Will. Their faith gave them tremendous poise and resilience needed for such difficult decisions.

VC's surgery was a very technically difficult one. Some of her huge cysts contained thick pus like fluid, and she developed pneumonia the day after surgery requiring to be put back on the ventilator. Her muscle mass was so poor that her respiratory muscles had become weak, making it difficult to wean her off the respiratory support for almost two weeks. She even developed cardiac arrest once but was immediately revived. Despite her challenges, VC came out victorious and was sent home after five weeks in hospital. God upheld the faith of her parents by giving them VC's unimaginable survival. She was back in her country by one year of age, celebrating her first birthday midair. Seven years down the line, VC remains well, free from any complications as testimony to the grace of the Universe and the power of human will.

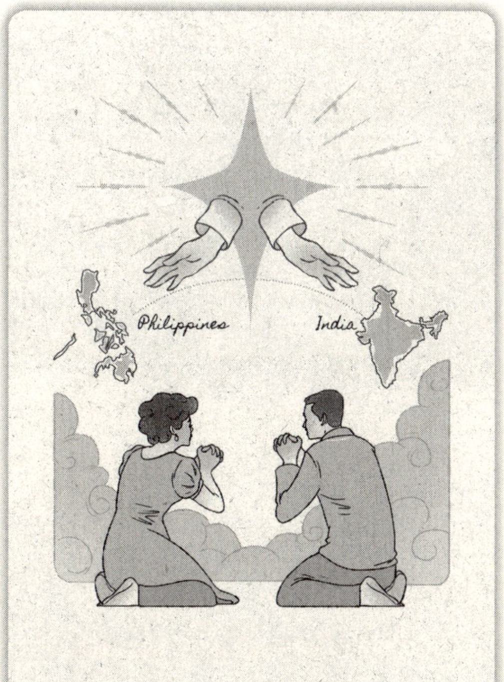

Clinical perspective:

VC was a very difficult case. Surgically very challenging as she had huge cysts that obscured and buried the porta and compressed the portal vein. Intraoperatively, the portal vein flow was present, and it had seemed blocked on scans due to the compression by the cysts. Few of the cysts contained turbid fluid that led to her septicemia and pneumonia that could have been life threatening considering her malnourished state. Her survival cannot be just attributed to the technical success of the operating techniques, because without the exemplary postoperative intensive care, her recovery was questionable. Despite a brief cardiac arrest, she has normal neuro-cognitive outcome. Her graft function is normal, and she has no late complications to date.

VC's success proved our mettle to the Filipino community, that then chose India in greater numbers as their destination for the surgery.

THE INVINCIBLE ONE

A young couple sat across us, with their almost four-year-old daughter in tow, in our specialist outreach clinic conducted monthly in Ranchi, Jharkhand to provide specialized medical consultation to children with liver and gastrointestinal diseases. Seemingly simple people of modest means—from a rural background and limited formal education—left us surprised and impressed with their quick comprehension, intelligence and prompt acceptance of the battery of investigations required for their little girl with liver disease.

Their daughter, Ruhani, was a quiet girl. She was very cooperative with her examination and didn't create any fuss when pricked for blood tests. She had a chronic liver disease with enlarged firm liver and deranged liver enzymes along with some degree of jaundice. The previous year, amidst the covid wave, she had developed chicken pox infection that had resulted in liver failure leaving her critical in the ICU for may days. Fortunately, she survived her first brush with death.

They were very regular and compliant with follow up visitations in the state monthly clinic for almost three months. She was diagnosed with autoimmune sclerosing cholangitis, characterized by inflammation in the liver and bile ducts caused by the body's immune system to act against its own liver and biliary system. An exceedingly rare disease that can be very devastating and progressive despite optimal therapy. Ruhani's liver was already severely damaged due to the indolent chronic disease activity, but in compensated state, where the complications of chronic failure had not set in. At every visit, Ruhani's father, who never refused any evaluation regardless of the cost, had only one persistent query, 'Nothing will happen to her, sure? She will be cured, won't she?' in his native tongue.

One day the father called us in panic to say that she had developed abdominal distension and her jaundice had increased. The realization that she hadn't responded to her treatment of immunosuppression and her liver was giving away left us with a burdened heart. They were called over to Delhi. An unfamiliar lady was accompanying Ruhani's father, but I brushed it away assuming my memory to be faulty. Medications were adjusted and the need for liver transplant for cure was discussed. An upper GI endoscopy was done that revealed high risk engorged varices and swollen blood vessels in the lower end of the food pipe (esophagus). This development happened due to increased pressure in the network of vessels supplying the liver by increasing resistance as the liver hardens with progressive disease. They would need ligation or else they could burst and cause life threatening bleeding. However, she also had severe extensive fungal infection in the esophagus that we decided to treat first to prevent its further spread in the body. A repeat endoscopy was scheduled for a week later. They patiently stayed for a week in Delhi and then visited me again in my chamber. This time, I enquired about the unfamiliar lady. Ruhani's father introduced her as Ruhani's 'senior mother'. Assuming her to be Ruhani's aunt, I couldn't help but marvel how close knit her family must be. Upon this visitation, I informed them that Ruhani would need an endoscopy to ligate her varices and then a liver transplant for her cure. The father needed only one assurance that no harm would come to his daughter. After a detailed session all risks and challenges were explained and endoscopy scheduled but then, they didn't turn up for it. Follow up calls were not responded to. The daunting challenge of liver transplant had scared them away!

Few days later, we decided to try to contact them again considering a salvageable life would be lost just because the parents were naïve and gullible. As they were not responding to our calls, we requested another colleague to get in touch. He was familiar with their local dialect and could explain to them the gravity of the situation in a language that they could connect to. With the advice reinforced in a more relatable manner, they promised to follow up in my next outreach clinic visit. And they did, but as luck would have it, Ruhani developed bleeding from her unaddressed varices, for want of an endoscopy, on the same day! She was hospitalized immediately and transfused blood and IV fluids and other therapies to arrest the bleeding and its complications urgently instituted. How we thanked our good sense for getting through to them despite their resistance! They stayed 200 km away from Ranchi and had they not been visiting the clinic that day, Ruhani would have bled to her death in her village! She now had survived her second brush with death!

Once stabilized, she was transferred to Delhi and was admitted for pretransplant optimization and evaluation. Fundraising needed to be instituted to bear the cost of her transplant. Her mother was the proposed donor. This time, both the women I had previously met were caring for Ruhani together like sisters. Curiosity took the better of me and I again enquired about her relation. Same answer 'senior mother'. Upon musing that she might be the brother-in-law's wife, they turned sheepish. It was then I realized that both the women were married to Ruhani's father!

He came over to our chamber the next day. In the process of caring for children with chronic diseases, clinicians come to develop a certain bond with their regular patients. So far, the man had come across as a very genuine trustworthy person of good values who stood by his family like a rock. When he spoke, he gave an insight and perspective that cannot come standing from the privileged lives of city dwellers. He had been married for eight years and when they could not have children, he married again as he desperately wanted a family. Holding back his tears, he said with defeat, 'I remarried to make a family. I have lost all I had trying to save Ruhani. All my resources are depleted, land sold off. All that remains is the humble roof on our head in our village. Nothing will happen to Ruhani, right, ma'am?'

We brushed all our judgements under the carpet. Who were we to judge a poor uneducated rural man struggling for his family? What access to IVF did he have back in his village? What were the social norms and taboos regarding adoption in his community? The enormity of the responsibility we were carrying on our shoulders had dawned on us … Ruhani had to be saved!

Blessings seemed to have dawned as support started arriving unexpectantly. The father of the child admitted on the adjoining bed in the multibed ward overheard the family's severe financial constraints and covered the entire bill of that hospitalization. Ruhani was stable and discharged, awaiting the donor evaluations, fund raising and participating in other preparations before a final date for her transplant would be decided. Funds were a trickle and slow to come through. As the family had already exhausted their resources, the entire cost would need to be raised through crowd funding and donations. Another of our patient's family put in a significant contribution. The family waited patiently, so did we, as Ruhani remained in a stable condition despite her advanced liver disease.

While awaiting transfer of the funds, her transplant had been scheduled for the ensuing week when catastrophe struck. Ruhani again developed variceal bleed despite the recent ligation and was admitted to the pediatric ICU. An emergency transplant was listed for the morning but overnight she worsened due to torrential bleeding. Her haemoglobin dropped to 3 gm/dl and her blood pressure started falling. She was put on a ventilator and an emergency very high-risk endoscopy was done in the night. The possibility of her dying on us was our biggest scare, as all that could be seen in the field of vision in her esophagus was oodles of blood. Despite the blinding, the bleeding varices were ligated, and in the middle of the procedure she vomited a massive amount of blood, and her sheets were all drenched red. Our hearts sank, we have perforated her stomach or esophagus we thought. It seemed like the end was close. We looked at the monitors, her vitals were better. With the accumulated clotted blood that we couldn't suction out cleared away by the huge vomitus, the insides could be seen clearly. All the bleeding points had been addressed and active bleed arrested. We literally jumped in joy as there was a chorus of celebratory chatter and laughter. Ruhani had survived her third brush with death!

The dawn would take her to the operation theatre for her transplant resulting in the culmination of all the efforts over the previous few weeks or so we thought as we went home that night. Man proposes, God disposes! Further trials were awaiting us as Ruhani's mother who was to be the donor tested covid positive. The transplant would have to be deferred for another week! Ruhani, too, developed pneumonia and fever and continued to be on a ventilator. Her father's words haunted us: 'Nothing will happen to Ruhani, right?'

Over the week as her mother recovered, so did Ruhani. She improved gradually and was removed from the ventilator. Her fever subsided. Though she continued to be sick on many parameters, we proceeded with the transplant, that was now very high risk, considering the recent severe complications. She had perhaps completed her share of troubles as the post-transplant recovery was as smooth as the rocky pretransplant course. She was discharged home in two weeks, a week earlier than her transplant package would be completed.

Having travelled back to their village, they follow up with her monthly blood test results telephonically with the message 'Your Ruhani is well'.

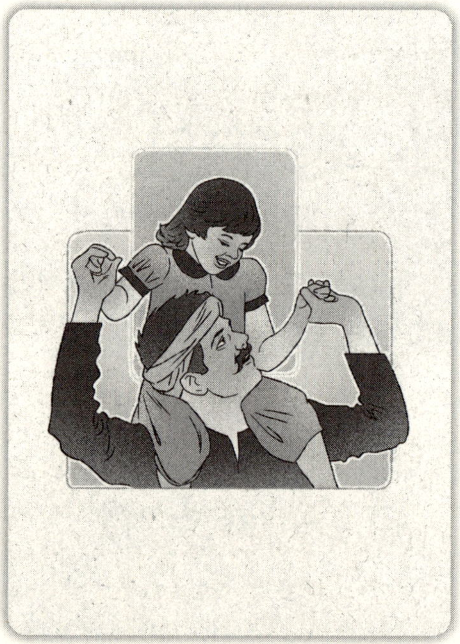

Clinical Perspective

This story represents the socio-cultural-economic challenges that we face trying to extend the reach of liver transplantation to the grass root level. A family that could not access infertility treatment managed to pull through a liver transplant only because we met them at their doorstep, held their hand and pulled them back to the medical fold when they had lost courage.

Her recent bleed and pneumonia that could have been due to covid (though she tested negative) as her mother was affected made her more fragile. With increasing experience, more and more complicated patients are being successfully transplanted despite other organ morbidities.

BAHUBALI

Bright red bangles, the 'chooda' young Punjabi women wear as a sign of new matrimony, still adorned her wrists as the young mother cradled her four-month-old jaundiced little boy, Ayush. Evaluations had revealed he had biliary atresia, a disease that was a death sentence half a century ago. Her once vibrant face had turned ashen, the joy of carefree youth replaced by the burden of maturity, responsibility and sacrifice. A few months down the line, he would need a liver transplant.

The enormity of the challenge daunted the young couple. They would need to arrange the funds required, win over the confidence of their parents and make arrangements to stay in Delhi for a few months to brace themselves for the forthcoming challenge. They resolved to save their first born, the mother offering to be the donor. They stuck to their decision even though their parents tried to dissuade them with concerns about short-term and long-term outcomes. They won over their trust and support with their sincerity and were very regular with his medications and followed all medical instructions. Another two to three months down the line, they would need to visit their transplant centre to kick in the process of fund raising and transplant optimization to enable a transplant; before he went into multiple complications of advancing liver disease.

A few weeks down the line, when they were ready with their tickets booked for the journey to Delhi, tragedy struck the simple middle class joint family, comprising of two brothers with their wives and children, and their parents. Ayush's uncle, his dad's brother, expired at the young age of thirty due to sudden myocardial infarction, leaving behind a young widow and two small children. The family was engulfed in grief, completely shattered by destiny's blow. Ayush's dad had suddenly aged, all responsibility now rested on his shoulders. A month flew by coping with the tragedy and life limping back to routine, and they then reached Delhi for the transplant evaluations.

His vaccinations were expedited, and the evaluations began. While the vaccine effects became robust in about three weeks, other preparations were duly made with donor and recipient tests. Funds had been arranged with the family pitching in about half of the cost and the rest through charity. A date for the surgery was about to be scheduled when Ayush's mother discovered she was pregnant! Embarrassed, disturbed and flustered by the unplanned conception the young couple went through a whirlwind of emotions! Despair, fear, guilt and concern for Ayush overwhelmed them; they could not rejoice in the prospect of welcoming a baby who in all probability would be healthy. They did not share the news with their elders fearing losing their support for the transplant. As it is they had had a difficult time countering their thought process of 'make another baby, why go in for transplant?' A baby inching towards death in her lap and another inching towards life in her womb, both could have a chance at life if another from the family would donate.

Alas that option was not explored! We never got a chance to persuade the father to come forward, as they came to us only after terminating the pregnancy. The transplant would have to wait approximately another three weeks before the mother would recover enough to be the donor. Despite the changing times, the onus of sacrifice still largely falls on the women in vast sections of our society, so painfully evident from the turn of events here!

Three weeks down the line, the surgery was finally scheduled. Ayush had a mild cough and cold, that didn't seem bothersome to us. However, his x-ray chest showed features of a viral pneumonia, and the transplant had to be deferred again! We would not get a clearance from the respiratory team for another week at least.

That week inched towards completion when Ayush became sick with fever and caught an infection that landed him in the ICU, something medical staff often fears of when awaiting transplants for babies. The lungs became worse than what they were with the virus previously and Ayush was on high end medications. He showed partial improvement but still was not clear of the infection, operating at this stage would entail high chances of an adverse outcome. We were on the lookout for a window when he would be stable enough to be taken up for the surgery. That window never came. Ayush deteriorated further, was on ventilatory support and in a condition most transplant centres would give up on.

The amount the family had saved for the transplant was almost exhausted in this critical phase. They now gave up on hope. It was very painful to see their predicament, a simple family of limited means who gave their all for their child—how would they reconcile to losing both their first born and their unborn baby who was sacrificed for him? What would they say to the skeptics who had prophesied they would waste time, money, effort, emotion and yet lose Ayush?

They came to us asking for a LAMA (leave against medical advice) as they could no longer pay for the ongoing ICU costs. They had given up, but we hadn't! Transplant was his only chance, and a new liver could steer him out of all the current complications, provided he survived the surgery. Mountain on one end and the deep sea on the other, it was an impossible choice but if the family would agree to donate despite the dismal chances, we were ready to take up the challenge. 'We must accept finite disappointment, but never lose infinite hope' said Martin Luther King Jr. That little hope in some corner of their hearts drove them to take their chance.

Magic happens when the universe sees truth and sincerity. Ayush was taken up for transplant on credit as a life saving measure, the shortfall in funds would be addressed later. The courage of the team and the parents paid off as Ayush, in that fragile state, withstood the twelve-hour surgery, healed through the days of post operative ventilation as his lungs gradually recovered and his new liver kicked in! He went home giving hope to the hopeless and immense confidence to us. A few months down the line during his routine follow ups, we marvel at his miraculous recovery. 'We call him "'Bahubali,"' said his parents, sheepishly referring to the larger-than-life character of the name in the blockbuster film *Bahubali*, who can brave it all.

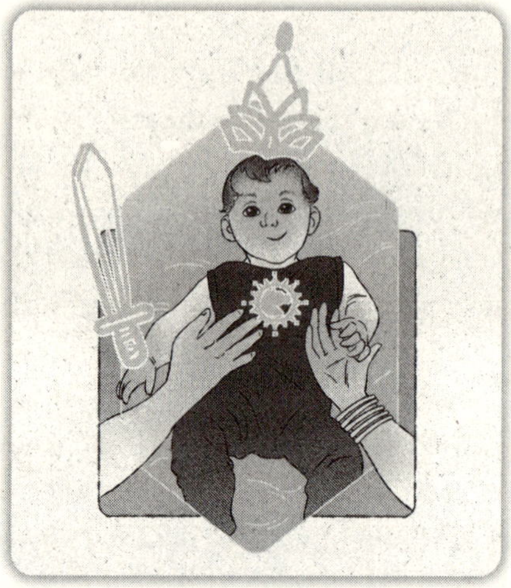

Clinical perspective:

Time is the most critical factor in babies with advancing liver disease. Timely intervention when severe complications have not yet set in minimizes suffering and costs, decreases both pre and post-operative hospital stay and improves outcomes. The diseases in these frail babies are ticking time bombs and at times, decisions made for their best interest may backfire. We deferred Ayush's transplant when his lungs were mildly affected only to transplant him later in a critical condition with pneumonia requiring him to be on a ventilator for days before and after the surgery.

It is a difficult situation, transplanting a very sick baby with a high chance of mortality when living donor transplant is being performed. Putting a donor through a major surgery when survival chances are not high is a huge moral dilemma, as is giving up on a baby who is holding and fighting for a chance at life.

NEVER SAY DIE

As the age old saying goes, 'Life is not a bed of roses.' For most it reflects on the struggles one goes through in building a life while fulfilling responsibilities. For a select few like Eli, taking birth itself seems to be a landing on a bed of thorns. How many in her predicament perish is difficult to enumerate, but her journey to survival is deeply humbling and exalting at the same time.

A fever and a fit, on day three of life, kept her in hospital for a month after her birth in her homeland, the Philippines. She had developed meningitis, an infection that causes swelling of the membranes covering her brain. It is a catastrophic infection that can lead to multiple sequelae, including loss of vision or hearing, limb weakness or seizure disorder and needs antibiotic therapy for minimum three weeks. Fortunately, Eli recovered well with an intact neurological outcome.

The young parents were now engrossed in looking after their firstborn who had become more precious, considering her criticality in her first month of life. A few weeks down the line they noticed her eyes were yellow and her tummy was becoming bigger. She was already five months old by the time evaluations were completed. She was diagnosed with biliary atresia. Delayed diagnosis results in missing the early window of three months; when a surgery can provide an opportunity for bile drainage to be achieved, and liver transplant delayed for a few months to years. Saddened that the early clues were missed, the parents gathered courage and began preparations for her eventual transplant.

Being a technical supervisor for live events like concerts and theatre, her father was able to mobilize crowdfunding and grants through some organizations for her treatment. They reached India when she was nine months of age, but she weighed only 3.6 kg, the ideal weight of a newborn! She would eat very little and was predominantly only breast fed. With her advanced disease, her malnutrition left her very vulnerable, and we immediately took her in for nutritional rehabilitation. A feeding tube was put in her stomach through her nostril to ensure adequate caloric and protein intake. With feeding optimized in a couple of days, we intended to send her home on tube feeding, but noticed she wasn't moving a leg that had also become swollen. Given the state of her fragile bones and nutritional status, we assumed it to be a fracture. It wasn't that simple though! She had developed osteomyelitis, i.e., infection of the bone that would require surgical debridement and antibiotic therapy for four to six weeks, if at all her failing liver would give her that much time! She braved through the surgery despite her marginal reserves and gradually recovered over the ensuing weeks. Friends and family furthered their crowdfunding efforts to sustain her additional costs of treatment, and it was another two months before her transplant could finally be scheduled.

On admission for the surgery, she was detected to have two fractures in her leg bones—one was recent and another already through partial stages of healing. A slab was applied to immobilize the limb and transplant performed as scheduled without further delay. The surgery went well, but on abdominal closure, the blood that flows through the veins would decrease due to abdominal compartment effect, i.e., effect due to increased pressure in the abdomen. Hence, an inlay mesh abdominal wall closure was done instead of a skin closure. Her post-operative course was stormy. An infection soon after the surgery requiring high-end antibiotics, respiratory issues requiring a chest tube, and many days of ventilation, skin complications at edge near mesh causing the wound to gape and requiring multiple dressings by the plastic surgeon, a redo surgery in the second week due to a leak, another fracture managed conservatively; the list was endless. She braved through each of them to be discharged on day thirty-four of the surgery only after celebrating her first birthday in the ICU!

She continued to recover well and gain weight after surgery. Her abdominal dressings continued and about six months down the line she was taken up for mesh removal, and a skin graft was inserted to close her abdomen. Her final step, too, had been successfully done and they would soon book tickets to return home. A day before departure, her liver enzymes showed some derangement, and the family cancelled their tickets. Covid was in force and health resources further drained, they didn't wish to take a chance.

The derangement settled with appropriate medication adjustments and little Eli continued to grow rapidly. She was now learning to stand. During this time, she fell during one of her attempts and fractured a leg again, requiring a cast for three weeks. A month later, all set to go with tickets rebooked, the parents were detected covid positive and they had to again stay back. It had already been over a year that they had been in India. Eli had celebrated her first birthday in the ICU, Diwali in an Indian shimmery lehenga, Christmas and New Year as well. She looked adorable as we walked into our OPD's, decked up in Indian attire and accessories along with the 'bindi' on her forehead. India had become her second home.

Finally, after about fourteen months here, they finally flew back to their country. Four years down the line, Eli continues to do well, and we keep receiving her videos as she achieves new milestones. Her parents run a TV show in her name that inspires families in similar predicaments. Words can't do justice to describe the commitment of her parents who are yet to plan another baby.

She has been one of our toughest cases; she is our trophy kid. One to never give up, never say die.

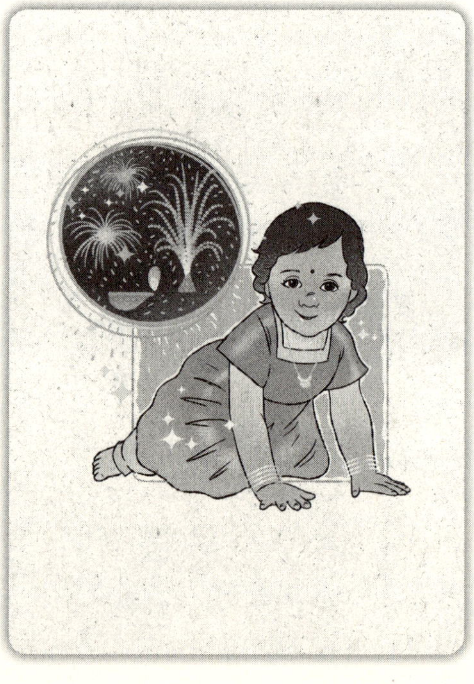

Clinical perspective:

Severe malnutrition and poor bone health are two very important factors that impact the recovery in liver transplant recipients. Eli's poor nutritional status made her vulnerable to the many complications she faced during her recovery. Her bones were so fragile that we feared that the pressure of the retractors used during the surgery would make them crack. Her abdomen was so small that she returned from the surgery with a gaping open abdominal wall without a covering of skin. The mesh that was placed was a constant threat as a potential source of infection. We had hoped that as she recovered and gained weight it would be possible to suture together her skin margins, but she required a skin graft. Her recovery through multiple medical issues over such a prolonged time-period was a great learning for us to never give up.

THE ABANDONED ONE

The complexities and intricacies of the human mind and heart that shape human behaviour is perhaps the most undecipherable language of the world. As health care providers, we get to watch closely in the most raw and unmasked form, the human response to adversity. As nonjudgmental as we may strive to become, there are many who leave us in awe and then there are those whom we can't comprehend the pain their decisions and actions inflict to their own. Khalil Ibrahim had said, 'Mother is the most beautiful word on the lips of mankind.' Perhaps, a mother's love is the only love that need not be deserved. Or should we say, a parent? The love and sacrifices of fathers are seldom talked about. Fatherhood is as much a privilege, profound responsibility and a state of unconditional love for one's offspring as motherhood has always been known to be. From a different perspective, have we glorified motherhood so much that a woman should cease to be one for herself once she begets a child? Drew Barrymore has said, 'Being a parent means loving your children more than you have ever loved yourself.' Human emotions are complex, what if a mother loves herself more than to wanting to live tending to a sick husband and child?

Hailing from West Bengal, Shauryadeep, lovingly called Shaurya, came to us in 2014 as an infant, almost eight months of age, due to his worsening jaundice and the itching that had set in. They had had multiple visits to various doctors ever since he was born before they were referred to us. We made a diagnosis of Alagille Syndrome, a genetic disorder that affects one in 30-50,000 infants and affects the excretion of bilirubin leading to jaundice, itching and damage to the liver. The severity of itching and progress of jaundice are variable, and they need regular monitoring of their liver function and modulation of medications to keep symptoms at bay. Shaurya's disease gradually progressed, and his itching kept getting worse, so much so that it affected his sleep. His mother was so overawed by his constant hospital visits, medications and persistent symptoms that she couldn't cope and decided to leave. Shaurya's father was left alone to look after his ailing five-year child. Fortunately, his father and brothers remained a pillar of strength for him.

As the itching became unmanageable and the liver functions further deteriorated, Shaurya's condition now necessitated a liver transplant. He was seven years of age by now and would not pull further for long without a new liver. Most living related liver transplants in children are performed with either of the parents as donors. His father, now a single parent, was keen to donate but he suffered from chronic kidney disease himself and was ineligible as a potential donor. We asked the family to look for another relative to be a donor, but no one came forward. We registered Shaurya as a candidate for cadaveric organ. Cadaver organs become available only occasionally in this part of India and for a child to get a liver is rare, given the huge waiting list for adults.

Cadaveric donations from brain dead children are rarer, making the situation quite grim and dismal. We had cared for him for so many years, watching him deteriorate without any probability of a transplant in sight was quite distressing.

Another huge roadblock was the financial situation of the family. His father manages a small shop, and he had depleted his meagre resources over the health care costs over the years. He had virtually no resources to afford a transplant. The poignant situation inspired us to go beyond the call of duty to help this brave man who was battling his own illness and loneliness, while fighting for his son. We are blessed to have the support of generous donors who help us every time we have a patient in need. We managed to raise funds for him with their magnanimous donations. We had the money in the kitty, but an organ was nowhere in reach. Nineteen months passed by, and Shaurya's condition became very fragile. He only had a few weeks before liver failure would take him away.

Opportunity came knocking soon, when a brave family decided to donate the organs of their child who was declared brain dead after a tragic accident. We decided to split the liver into two halves. As Shaurya weighed only 17 kg, he would get the left lobe and an adult patient the right lobe. Shaurya was immediately flown in from Kolkata and wheeled into the operating theatre within twelve hours.

Shaurya did go through some post operative and some delayed complications but recovered well and has been doing well a few years down the line. Caring for another over our own self is only what makes us human. Perhaps it's a wiring for evolution as a few months ago Shaurya's dad succumbed to kidney failure. Shaurya continues to grow well in the loving care of his grandparents. Shaurya is all they have to live for now.

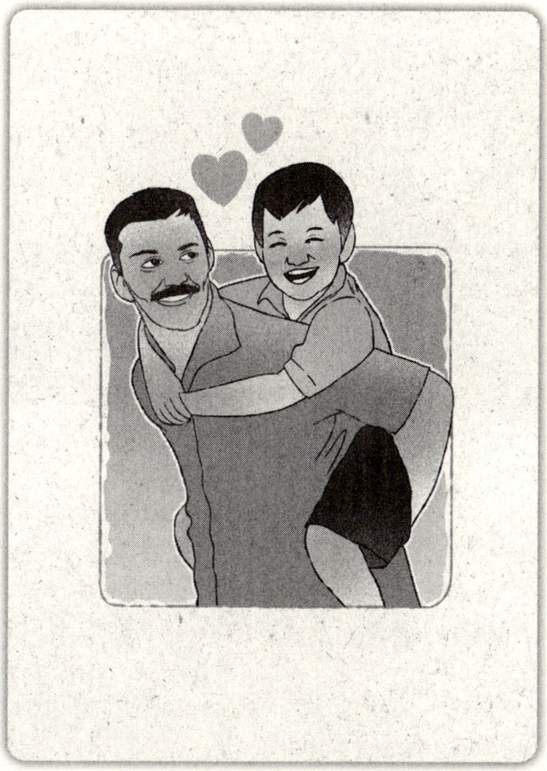

Clinical perspective:

Deceased organ donation is still very rare in our country especially in Northern India. There are countless who are lost for want of an organ. Fear of living donation and non-acceptance of cadaveric donation for various beliefs and reasons are the biggest stumbling blocks in saving many other lives.

ULTIMATE MEASURE YET ULTIMATE FAILURE

The human spirit has an unwavering ability to overcome. Only those who confront unusual challenges can flaunt and rejoice in unusual successes. For some, just being alive is their unusual success that sets benchmarks for those facing similar predicaments. 'Where there is a will, there is a way' is the motto for those who choose strength in adversity, this strength may be found in the humblest of souls.

Hundreds throng the specialty outpatient clinics at premier government institutes of the capital from all over the country. Children with various chronic liver diseases that may or may not improve with medications are amongst the cohort cared for by the pediatric hepatology services. Sadly, many of these disorders linger on for months and years, and many are lost to various complications. Ahmad, a little boy from an impoverished family from Bihar, suffered from a rare bile acid transporter defect that occurs in only about one in 50,000 to one in 1,00,000 children. Insights into this disease entity have emerged mostly in the last decade and it was expected that Ahmad's condition would progress rapidly in the early years of life causing progressive jaundice, intense itching, growth faltering and eventually liver failure.

The parents were very meticulous and ideal caregivers for Ahmad—very regular with their follow ups despite the distance, high travel costs along with loss of workdays, very particular with the medications despite their illiteracy. As the itch set in a diversion surgery, that often helps ameliorate the itching and delay the disease progress, was done at the premier institute. After a few months respite, the symptoms were back in full fury and Ahmad suffered from intense intractable itching. A liver transplant was the only treatment.

The first day we saw them in our clinic will remain etched in our memories. Ahmad's father, a frail thin man, sat with his itching equally frail four-year-old son in his lap. They hadn't slept soundly for days as Ahmad was constantly itching. His yellow skin had thickened, darkened and bruised all over with scratch marks. Their relatively well-off relatives in Delhi had brought them to us after their institute told them about our subsidized transplant program. One of Ahmad's aunts was a graduate who discussed the situation with us. She would become the single consistent force that catalyzed Ahmad's transformation.

Ahmad's blood group matched with his father. 'Will I be able to pull my cart after the donor surgery?' 'Will I be able to lift a sack on my shoulders?' were questions no potential donor had ever asked us. He sold daily-use small time plastic goods on his cart for his living. Here was a man who could hardly earn enough to feed his family, the sole breadwinner of a large one. We come across many people who withhold and conceal their resources to get financial aid and feign lack when there isn't. Here was this man who was willing to work beyond his capacity, stretch his means to partially meet the costs, while seeking funding as the lakhs needed were beyond his reach. His grace, humility, and dignity of conduct despite his misery deeply inspired us to help them.

Funds were raised through crowdfunding, NGOs, and individual donors to cover the cost of his subsidized transplant. With his new liver, he recovered rapidly. The itching was gone and the frowning, cranky, irritable and quick-to-anger child transformed into an exuberant and excited boy with tantrums and demands. They had stayed a long time in Delhi due to the illness. Often, the ones with the humblest of means have the largest hearts to share. Their relatives remained a constant source of support for them and Ahmad's aunt was by their side all along. The family moved to Delhi and Ahmad's dad resumed his work here. A bag full of clips, hair bands, safety pins and other knick-knacks that he sold, was brought for us as a thank you gift!

The follow up care was provided jointly by our team and the referring institute. Their regular scheduled monitoring tests and medications were taken care of by their institute. A few weeks later, Ahmad's liver function tests become deranged, and he was detected to have a biliary stricture, a complication that may occur in up to 20 per cent liver transplant recipients. He would require endoscopic stent placement. The family was resolute and without an iota of complaint. Additional costs were entailed and despite being a strain for the family, they never appeared flustered, hostile or frustrated. Ahmad underwent the procedure four times at intervals of a few months, all as a free patient.

He transformed into a handsome kid, unrecognizable from his pre transplant persona. As his skin healed, it softened, and the texture improved. With catch up growth, he rapidly gained in weight, height and energy. His sister who dropped out of college due to the physical and financial demands of caring for him, resumed her studies. All through his follow ups, it was only the women in the family who brought him along, as his dad earned their daily living from his cart. He has stood up and proved how right Martin

Luther King Junior was when he said, 'The ultimate measure of a man is not where he stands in moments of comfort and convenience, but where he stands at times of challenge and controversy.'

The greatest achievements can also become the bedrocks of the greatest failures. There are only anecdotal case reports of disease recurrence after transplant for Ahmad's condition. One of our biggest success stories became our most painful loss when Ahmad developed symptoms again. It is so rare that initially we just tried to exclude other complications like rejection and stricture recurrence. He was again jointly cared for at our hospital and the initial referring institute who managed his recurrence very well and his jaundice and itching were again controlled. The family continued to toil with regular visits and enhanced treatments till one day Ahmad developed a rapidly progressive fatal infection that took him away within a few hours very recently.

There is a power greater than you and I are, the Ultimate that belittles our ultimate for reasons human mind cannot decipher.

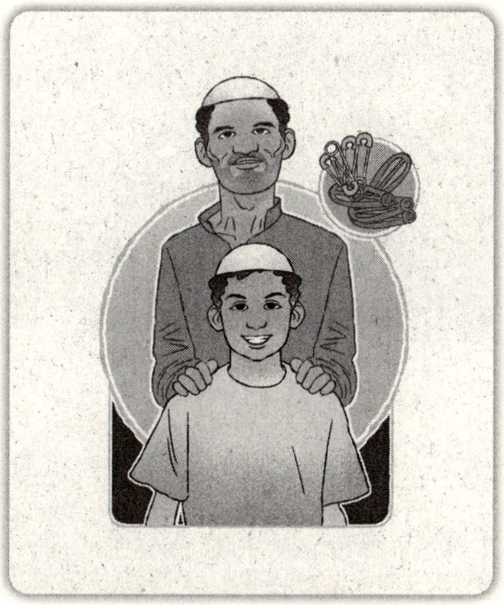

Clinical perspective:

Ahmad got very good care at the referring institute and the joint care provided resulted in his recovery. Confidence building from the primary care team, timely referral, and patient ownership with special interest on follow up, made his survival from a devastating disease possible. It took months for his skin to attain a normal texture and for his growth to catch up. The biliary stricture was well managed with ERCP and stent placements; replacements that very few have competency for in small children.

He was restored to normal health and had a disease-free life for a few years. Disease recurrence, exceedingly rare, too was managed very well back at the referring institute. The therapies required predispose to severe infections and that's what we lost him to.

WHAT IS IN A NAME?

'What is in a name?' Skeptics believe it's irrelevant, astrology and numerology swear by its influence and many philosophies consider it to shape or define one's personality. Whatever made the young couple choose to name their first born Demir, meaning as strong as iron, his life made him prove himself worthy of his name right in his toddlerhood.

Born in Kashmir to a beautiful young couple, he was a gift of joy to them. His light-colored twinkling naughty eyes enraptured his adoring mother who took a break from her engineering career to bring him up. He started playschool in his third year, and she was contemplating returning to her profession when they were pulled into a journey of pain and deep suffering that changed them forever.

Demir was passing red colored urine that was initially thought to be due to a urine infection. As it recurred in the ensuing weeks, further tests were done, and the family moved to Chandigarh for his evaluations. He was found to have a mass in his left kidney that proved to be a Wilms' tumour, the most common cancer of the kidneys in children, that usually affects those less than five years of age. Demir underwent sessions of chemotherapy, before being operated for removal of his affected kidney, followed by multiple sessions of radiotherapy. Demir's chemotherapy sessions left him sick, and he later developed a severe skin rash due to the radiotherapy. Their battle with cancer was a painful journey that left scars on their psyche that gnawed to the core, their cheerful selves became subdued into a quiet persona. Gradually life limped back to normal over the ensuing weeks and Demir began to regain his cheerful self. He had begun his second stint at life.

As though cancer was not enough to test his mettle, life very cruelly threw another volley at him with a force so fearful that it almost took him away. Demir was three and a half when he developed fever, vomiting and belly ache that progressed, and he also became jaundiced. He was hospitalized in their hometown and doctors hoped he would recover in a few days as most children with viral hepatitis do. However, tests for usual viruses that affect the liver were negative, and his jaundice continued to deepen. A week passed and Demir became aggressive with markedly agitated behaviour—an ominous sign in liver disease. It reflects brain dysfunction due to advanced liver failure and carries very high risk to life. Demir's parents were told he hardly had any chance and was advised to put Demir on a ventilator in the intensive care unit. Had he gone through the agony of cancer chemotherapy, surgery and radiation only to die of liver failure in a few months? His parents were devastated.

Their doctors told them that shifting him to a higher centre of care might give him a chance. His parents reached out to us via a tele-consult, and we advised them that he needed to be put on a ventilator and airlifted in an air ambulance as early as possible. Faced with the prospect of losing their child, they decided to move but were daunted by the need to ventilate. They could not afford an air ambulance and chose to travel in an ambulance by road without ventilatory support. Their journey would take them about twenty four hours, with limited compromised care during travel that would further worsen his condition and was not medically advisable. They had no choice; their child was dying.

They reached us a day later and Demir was immediately put on a ventilator and dialysis was started to remove ammonia from his body that had been accumulating because of his failing liver and causing increased pressure in his brain. This high pressure that had been present over the previous forty-eight to seventy-two hours could cause irreversible brain damage. His mother's blood group matched, and her donor evaluations were started immediately. In less than twenty-four hours, he was wheeled into the operation theatre after thorough evaluations including a CT scan of his brain to ensure he had no irreversible brain damage that would preclude his recovery from the coma.

As Demir recuperated post liver transplant and his new liver functioned well, he began to open his eyes and try to move his limbs. He continued to be on a ventilator, awaiting full regaining of his consciousness. He was awake and breathing on his own when he was finally removed from the ventilator after only about a week. Though conscious, he was not able to follow commands, interact and speak. One of the veins to the liver developed a clot and he underwent an angiography procedure to remove it and dilate the vein. The procedure was successful, and his liver and abdomen were improving. Neurologically, he continued to be in a noncomprehensive state. Demir was back, but was he?

MRI brain showed swelling over some parts of the brain and appropriate medications were instituted. His parents were deeply disturbed, would Demir live only to be lost in an unknown state of his consciousness? Days passed and he remained the same. No response, no words, no interaction. Medication doses were further hiked, and he was discharged awaiting his neurological recovery, the extent and timing of which were unpredictable. He had been wheeled in on a stretcher, was discharged on a wheelchair with a heavy heart.

Days and weeks passed and slowly and steadily he showed marked improvement. His liver parameters remained stable, and he began to comprehend, respond and speak. Six months down the line, he walked into our outpatients and breezed into our hearts with his chatter! His neurological recovery was remarkable thanks to the plasticity of the growing brain in children. The family was happy and content that they were finally out of the woods. His mother discussed her plans to resume her career as we enthusiastically encouraged her.

Life was not done testing Demir's strength though. A few weeks later his mother called in to say that Demir had been having fever on and off for a month. Aghast, we referred them to our colleagues in their city and he was detected to have a large pneumonia affecting his left lung. He was hospitalized but there was no response to adequate antibiotics and his respiratory status worsened over the next two days. He was rushed to us on oxygen support and further evaluations reveal his Wilms' tumor has relapsed into his lung! With chemotherapy, his oncologist was very hopeful that he had about 70 per cent chance of recovery. He needed all the strength his name conferred on him to make that chance work and work it did. He is tumour free and doing perfectly well on follow-up, lungs, liver, brain et al!

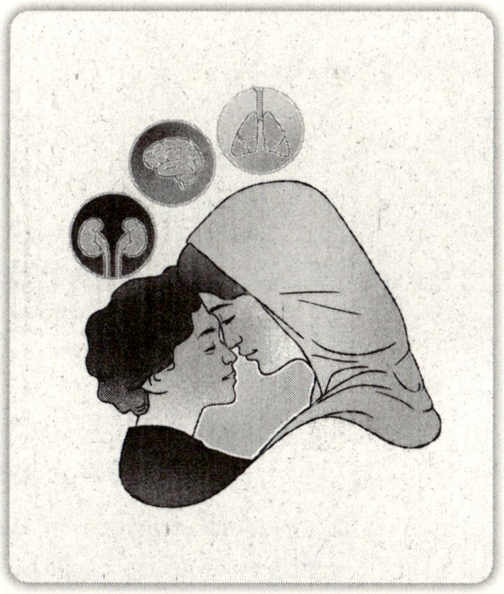

Clinical perspective:

Liver transplant in acute liver failure is a race against time requiring timely diagnosis, early referral, appropriate transport, good intensive care and transplant before multiorgan failure or severe brain damage sets in. Transferring to a liver unit needs an air ambulance which has issues with affordability and logistics. Early ventilation is neuroprotective but transporting a child on ventilator by a road ambulance over a long distance is difficult. The prolonged neurological morbidity in Demir might have been minimized if the transport had not been so challenging.

Tumour-relapse that may occur post-transplant pushes the patient back into the grind of hospitalizations and repeated therapies that often shatter the morale of families facing the transplant challenge.

INDIVIDUAL DESTINIES

What is destiny? Believers in destiny are of the firm view that a destiny designed by God can never be changed by man. How else can one comprehend the contrasting destinies of two children born in the same family? Does destiny influence what we call fate? Or it is just a reflection of our inadequacies, that we fail to provide equal opportunities to all in our families or say society by large?

As clinicians and health care providers, we get to closely watch what illness unfolds for people and how it impacts their very essence. There are a few that leave us deeply affected and remain etched in our memories. The tale of Anushka's family is one of them.

A resident of Bihar, Anushka, the eldest of three children, was nine years old when she developed jaundice. When it did not improve with their primary care doctor's treatment, she was referred to a premium institute in Patna where her evaluations revealed she had Wilson's disease. Wilson's disease is an inherited disorder in which copper accumulates in the body in several organs, mainly the liver and brain. This accumulation occurs gradually, and the child may not develop symptoms at all till it becomes advanced. Anushka's liver was already quite damaged and shrunken by the time her disease was discovered. She was further referred to a premier institute in Delhi where she remained hospitalized for many days. She was started on medications that would help chelate the excess copper from her body. She also underwent multiple sessions of plasma exchange to rapidly lower the copper load from her body. The treatments helped and she began to improve. She was discharged on medications hoping that despite her severely damaged liver, copper chelation would prevent further damage, and she would remain in a compensated stage of chronic liver disease.

A few weeks down the line, Anushka deteriorated suddenly and was immediately readmitted to her institute in Delhi. Over the span of a few hours, she became very critical. She had developed acute liver failure with encephalopathy, i.e., brain dysfunction due to the increased pressure in the brain as a result of retained metabolites; the sick liver couldn't help the body. This is a devastating scenario as acute liver failure in Wilson's disease is known to be universally fatal without a liver transplant. Anushka needed a new liver as soon as possible if she had to live. In countries that have robust cadaveric liver donation programs, she would be on the top priority list and an organ would be allocated to her as soon as one became available from a braindead donor. Liver transplantation for children in India is still largely provided by the private sector and is living donor related.

Anushka's treating team reached out to us asking for the feasibility of an urgent transplant. The parents had already drained their resources in her treatment so far. A rural agriculture based joint family with her father in a small-time job in Delhi, they were in no position to afford a liver transplant, that too at such a short notice.

Moreover, her blood group was not compatible for donation with that of her parents. Though blood group incompatible transplants are now being increasingly performed, they are more challenging requiring special expensive medications and treatments and carry a higher risk of complications. Fortunately, we had some corpus fund that we had raised for other patients which went unused as the intended recipient passed before they could undergo the transplant planned for them. We had the money; her mother was willing to donate. A blood group incompatible transplant in acute liver failure is amongst the most challenging scenarios for us. We decided to take on the challenge.

Anushka was shifted to us, and she was immediately put on a ventilator and dialysis started—measures that are protocol in such patients to minimize brain injury and prevent irreversible brain damage. Donor and recipient evaluations were started on a war footing and medications to bring down her antibodies, ones which would react with the incompatible-blood-group donated liver, given. Meanwhile she deteriorated further with her falling blood pressures, and she required medications to maintain her blood circulation. It was a race against time that we won. She was wheeled into the OT and in less than thirty six hours of presenting to us, she had undergone the transplant and come off her ventilator. Her miraculous destiny continued to propel her to further recovery and her new liver kicked in well. She went home in seventeen days.

As Wilson's disease is a genetic disorder due to a copy of diseased genes being inherited from each parent who are carriers, her siblings were screened but detected to be unaffected. Anushka developed a biliary stricture, a narrowing of the bile ducts where they are joined together at surgery, that was successfully addressed with an endoscopic dilatation and stent placement which was subsequently removed. She remains asymptomatic now and has resumed her schooling.

Life can be very cruel at times. Acute liver failure, a disease that happens less than one in a 1,00,000 struck the family again. A year down the line, we received a call again from the same team that had contacted us for Anushka. Her brother was in intensive care due to acute liver failure caused by acute Hepatitis A, a virus that affects the liver. Most patients with acute Hepatitis A suffer for a few days with pain abdomen, vomiting, poor appetite and jaundice before recovering over a few days to weeks. Less than 1 per cent of those affected by Hepatitis A develop acute liver failure. Anushka's brother was on ventilator, undergoing dialysis and receiving good intensive care. As he did not have any known underlying chronic illness, it was hoped that given a few days his liver may start recovering naturally. However, he continued to deteriorate, and a liver transplant emerged again as the only life-saving option.

We were very pained to learn about these tragic developments and were more than willing to help. Though we did not have any reserve funds this time, we were confident we could raise the desired amount from generous donors in a short time. We are very fortunate to be connected to philanthropic individuals with kind hearts who are just a call away to bail us out in such dire circumstances. Sadly, the family could not identify a donor this time. Anushka's mother had already been a donor. Families dependent on single earning male members tend to be very scared of putting them through donor surgery, fearing loss of life or livelihood due to feared complications. A safe donor experience in the family was also not suffix for them to overcome that fear, and no donor came forward. Her brother died the death her mother and our team had saved Anushka from.

As we celebrate and rejoice in Anushka's miracle every time she visits us in the outpatients, a thought of her brother, who was not as fortunate, always creeps in. It is our society's failure that parents who love their daughters no less, as exemplified by their going all out to save Anushka, feel insecure without a male child. Despite having Anushka and her sister, the loss of their only son has made them plan another child, hoping he will come back to them. Anushka's mother, who has gone through 3 childbirths and a donor surgery, is now carrying another child—her pregnancy is further testimony to donor safety that we wish more men understood.

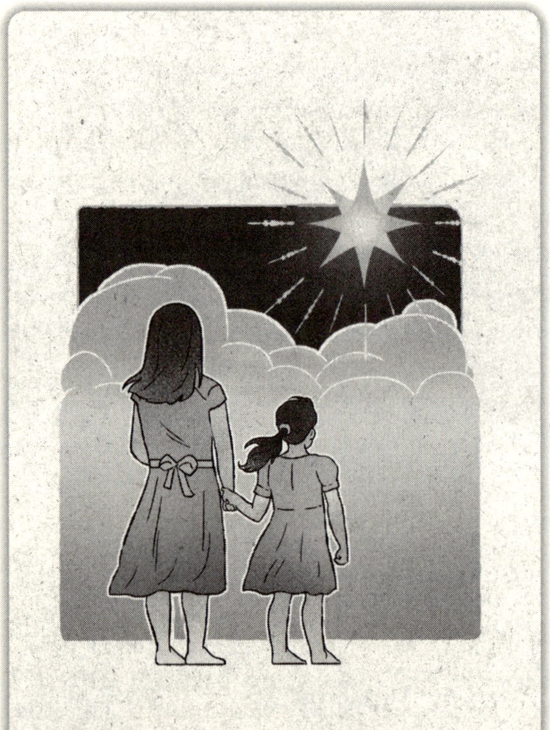

Clinical perspective:

Fulminant liver failure is an exceedingly rare condition. Why some children with the same illness have a slower and milder course while other few develop ALF needs further study. Though the genetic evaluation did not pick up any aberration, perhaps, both siblings had some predisposing factor that medical science has yet to decipher.

Though successful living donor transplants have now been performed in the country for twenty five years with safe donor experience, concerns with donor safety are still a major roadblock. The dire need to promote cadaveric donations can no less be emphasized.

DOUBLE WHAMMY

'If you want the rainbow you must put up with the rain,' the famous quote flashes up in the mind whenever this family visits us for their follow ups in the outpatients. A happy couple with their two young sons, all four with a striking similarity in their body physique and their ever smiling and cheerful persona. They share a unique, remarkable and highly inspiring common thread that speaks volumes of their strength through a very challenging common destiny. A simple middle class single income family from a city in UP, each member has a scar of liver surgery on their tummies. Both the parents have been liver donors for their sons who both are chronic liver disease survivors saved by successful liver transplants!

Their younger son Kishan was only eight months old when during a diarrheal episode, his doctor noticed an enlarged spleen on examining him. Further evaluations revealed he had portal hypertension, i.e., elevated pressure in the portal venous system that drains blood from the stomach, intestines, pancreas and spleen into the liver for filtration before reaching the heart and back into the body circulation. When the liver is diseased and scarred, blood flows through the portal vein against resistance leading to increased back pressure, enlarged and tortuous collateral veins in the food pipe and rectum that may rupture to cause life threatening bleeding. Kishan underwent a liver biopsy and was diagnosed to have congenital hepatic fibrosis, a genetic developmental disorder resulting in abnormal development of the portal veins and bile ducts, leading to progressive liver scarring, portal hypertension and eventually over the years liver cirrhosis and chronic liver failure.

Kishan now needed regular visits to his pediatric gastroenterologist, based in Delhi, for regular surveillance endoscopies to check for and ligate any abnormal enlarged veins in his food pipe. His father worked in a pharmaceutical company and was very diligent and regular with the scheduled endoscopies that were initially required every few weeks and then at intervals of a few months. After a few months in the private sector, they chose to follow up at a premier government institute. Six years down the line, Kishan's brother Vidit, who was three years older to him, was also detected to have an enlarged spleen and portal hypertension due to congenital hepatic fibrosis. Both the brothers now remained under treatment of the same unit requiring periodic endoscopic procedures. Fortunately, none of the brothers had kidney involvement, that may also be part of the disease.

A year down the line, at eleven years of age, Vidit's liver began to give way and decompensate. His growth became affected and then he developed jaundice and ascites, i.e., fluid accumulation in the belly. He would now need a liver transplant, and they then came to us. His mom would be the donor. The dad had the economic responsibility of looking after his parents and his wife's mother, who all stayed with them, in addition to taking care of two children with chronic liver disease. Financial support was needed, his company bore half the cost of the transplant surgery, the rest was covered through crowd funding and by the family. Vidit recovered well.

Covid arrived, disrupting the regular endoscopic surveillance for their younger son. For almost two years the family did not visit hospital fearing contacting covid. Vidit remained well and his periodic blood tests remained in range, our inputs provided telephonically. With one child on immunosuppression post-transplant and another with chronic liver disease, they had an intense fear of catastrophe due to covid. This fear made them overlook the risk of bleeding due to portal hypertension; resulting in rapid deterioration in his liver that was in a compensated state. Kishan was brought to us in a sick state. He had had blood-streaked stools, developed lethargy and deep jaundice. He was detected to have infection and was very fragile. Any further deterioration could land him in the ICU. We were very distraught. Often , families reach us late due to ignorance and inability to recognize early signs of complications, something that did not hold true with them. We already had one post liver transplant patient, Anushka, who had lost a sibling to liver failure for want of a donor. Kishan's dad was willing to donate, but had a fatty liver and needed to lose weight before his liver could be accepted as a healthy donor graft. The boys had just three years between them and were just like twins, the guilt of failing one of them would be a burden they could not live with. Their predicament was very heart rendering for us as a team as well, and we hoped and prayed Kishan would live till his transplant became feasible.

Even in our imperfections, great things are accomplished with God's help. A higher force was witness to the family's efforts for Kishan ever since he was eight months old. Their courage was rewarded as we were able to tide over this phase as Kishan recovered from the infection and did not develop any catastrophic major bleed. His disease, however, was now very advanced and he was just giving us a window of opportunity to take him up for transplantation. His father took up a strict diet and exercise regimen, over a few weeks his liver fat parameters optimized. Alongside, he was busy making financial arrangements for the transplant. Provisions for a long leave for a few months could not be made as his job required lots of travelling and field work and he could not commit when he would be able to resume his duties. He now became jobless and could not seek financial help from the company as well. They ran a 'do-it-yourself' fundraiser amongst acquaintances and colleagues but not much could be raised.

Fortunately, they had a medical insurance for Kishan that covered the cost of the hospitalization episode before transplant and about a third of the transplant expenses. The rest of the cost was borne by the family. Kishan recovered well after his transplant though he did require endoscopic procedures for biliary stricture that resolved thereafter.

Four months down the line, his father was fit to resume work. With a kind consideration towards his circumstances, his company chose to cover these four months as nonpaid leave, and he was accepted back to continue his job. A fitter and happier self, he awaits partial reimbursement of his transplant expenses from his company. Meanwhile, Vidit, who needs tonsillectomy for his markedly enlarged tonsils awaits his time as his less urgent medical needs took a backseat during Kishan's transplant journey.

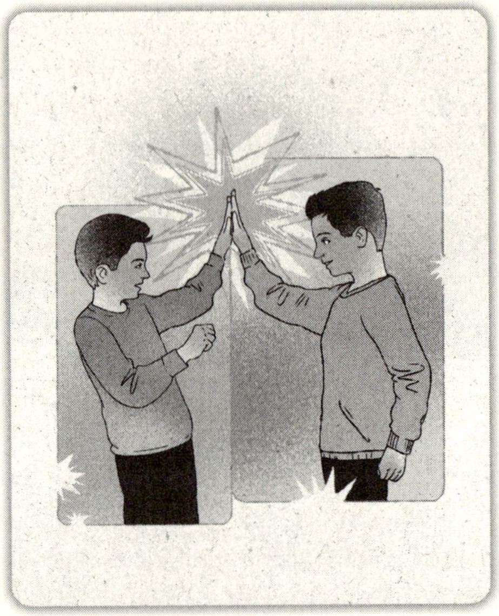

Clinical perspective:

More than one child may be affected in genetically transmitted disorders, especially when the disease manifests and is diagnosed later, precluding prenatal testing in next pregnancy. The socioeconomic implications are huge as they push the families to the edge and many a time, the investment required in terms of money, effort, mental strength, social support, career compromise, physical sacrifice of organ donation, and ongoing demands of post-transplant care may be so daunting that families find it difficult to choose the transplant option. Doing so twice over is truly remarkable. Both parents having compatible blood groups for donation is also not always the case. In the over 500 transplants in children at our centre, this is the only case where both siblings received a living donor liver transplant.

HE AIN'T HEAVY, HE'S MY BROTHER

'He ain't heavy, he is my brother' goes the famous song by the Hollies, the ballad inspired by a James Wells quote written in the late nineteenth century. The picture of a boy carrying another on his back became the logo with these words as its motto for the Boys Town, a refuge centre for homeless boys in the city of Omaha in the early twenthieth century. It was inspired by these words coming from an inmate, who would happily carry another polio ridden one with braces on his back up the stairs. It has since then come to symbolize the human spirit of enduring pain and discomfort for the sake of someone we care for. This spirit of taking on another's burden without considering otherwise is what makes families and true friends, and this is what has made living donor liver transplantation feasible. At some point in our lives, most of us have needed to be carried by someone, metaphorically speaking. And, at some point, we probably carried somebody else. We're human. We face challenges. And we look to each other for help when we do.

Aarti was the firstborn of a young couple in their early twenties. Hailing from a family from UP, Aarti's father is the eldest of three brothers living in a joint family set up with their parents. The brothers run a small-time grocery shop together. Aarti was welcomed with great cheer as the brothers had always missed having a sister. She was a cute little bundle of joy for the family, the 'Laxmi' of the house. The cheer soon turned to worry as a few days later she was noticed to be jaundiced. As it persisted and deepened, they visited multiple clinics and hospitals for her treatment with no respite. After running her through various levels of evaluations after being referred to a specialized government institute, she was finally detected to have biliary atresia and advised a Kasai surgery when she was barely four months of age. The parents had by now realized Aarti had a serious and grave diagnosis, and the results of the surgery was not very promising at this age. Seeing little hope, they wisely decided against it.

Another few weeks down the line as the disease progressed, Aarti's growth began to falter, her tummy became bloated due to fluid accumulation, enlarged liver and spleen, and she had intermittent fever spikes. At this stage, she was referred to us at almost seven months of age for a liver transplant. The parents were very confused and skeptical as they had heard various misconceptions about the procedure but were determined to save their little girl. We explained to them about transplantation, its challenges as well as the successes. They met a few of our post-transplant patients and their families, leading to their confidence in the modality and in us.

Aarti's medications and nutrition were optimized, and vaccinations expedited. The family could no way afford a transplant and would be able to chip in only about a third of the cost. Crowdfunding campaign was started, and NGOs approached for grants. Both her parents had blood groups compatible with hers and were willing to donate. Her father's evaluations began but he was rejected as a donor due to unfavourable anatomy. Aarti's mother underwent screening tests to assess her as a potential donor. To our surprise and dismay, the young lady who had no symptoms apart from an occasional cough, was suffering from tuberculosis in her lungs. Had she not had her evaluations, it would have gone undetected for longer until severe potentially life-threatening complications set in. She was referred to our chest specialists and appropriate treatment instituted. Aarti was also screened and when found free of the disease, started on prophylactic medication to prevent her from contacting tuberculosis from her mother. The medication is known to cause derangement in liver functions and with her precarious state, it was a very narrow road to trudge.

By now Aarti had continued to worsen, she had not gained weight despite our dietary interventions and weighed less than 5 kg. She developed fever and black tarry stools suggestive of bleeding in her stomach. She was hospitalized and treatments instituted. She had features of advanced portal hypertension but any therapeutic endoscopic intervention in her state was wrought with huge risk. If she bled catastrophically, we would have to take that risk, but thankfully the bleeding was controlled with conservative measures. We had put in a nasogastric tube for feeding to ensure adequate caloric intake for weight gain. Due to inadequate response, parenteral nutrition was instituted to provide nutrition through intravenous route.

The fever ravaged with no response to high end antibiotics that were upgraded step wise to maximal potency. Her blood culture grew a fungus and antifungal therapy was started. The IV-nutrition had to be discontinued as the fat content in it might perpetuate the infection. Her condition further worsened, and she was shifted to the ICU due to poor respiratory status. With no donor available, how far would she go even if we were able to tide over the current situation? We feared the family would opt out of further treatment. There was no donor, the money for the transplant they had was already exhausted, and she was not responding to the current medications. The parents were crestfallen.

Aarti's uncle, her father's younger brother, who was just twenty-three years of age came forward to be the donor. Her crowdfunding campaign had touched a nerve, won over hearts and funds poured in, so much so that we had a surplus despite her prolonged hospital stay. She was screened for any focus of fungal growth in her heart or brain, and another antifungal was added and other therapies intensified. To the joy of all, she responded and was out of the ICU in two days. Finally, her fever started to break, and her weight began to improve. She was in hospital for over a month before her cultures finally became sterile and she was taken up for a transplant. There was no looking back thereafter, and after another month in hospital she went back home leaving behind a legacy of hope and grit.

Five years down the line, she is a beautiful young girl who is the darling of the family and her medical team. She calls her uncle, who was her liver donor, her younger father who dotes on her and on her infant younger brother.

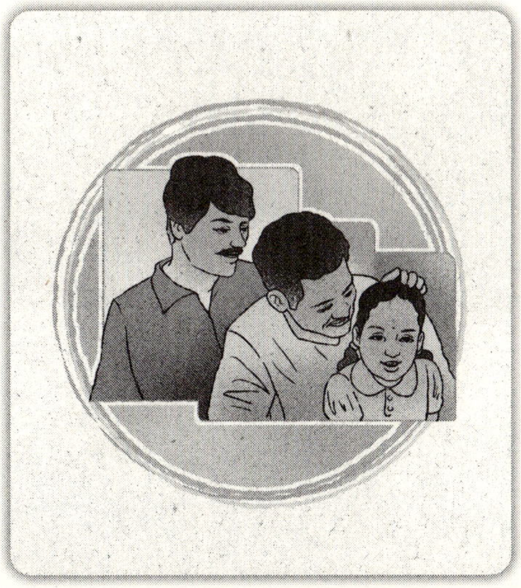

Clinical perspective:

Poor weight gain, infections and bleeding are amongst the most common problems we face in babies awaiting a liver transplant. Fungal septicemia is ominous with high risk to life, more so, in the setting of chronic liver failure. It may seed various organs and if not adequately eradicated flare up post-transplant as immunosuppression is instituted. This may happen despite negative cultures. Aarti was continued on antifungals after the surgery for a few days and thankfully, she remained free of systemic sepsis in her recovery phase.

We do have quite a few liver donors who are barely into adulthood. Choosing to be a liver donor so early into their youth calls for a lot of courage. Laparoscopic donor surgeries are now being increasingly performed to prevent the big scar of donor hepatectomy and its attendant body image issues.

ACKNOWLEDGEMENT

Our cultural ethos entwines us in the concept of destiny and karma. We would like to begin by thanking the universe and our shared destinies that led us to this profession, brought us together, and considered us worthy enough to be the channels of the Divine healing energy because 'We treat, He heals.'

It was the vision of our Chairman, Padam Vibhushan Dr Prathap C Reddy, to bring healthcare of international standards within reach of every individual giving us our 'karm bhoomi.' Dr Reddy's legacy has been carried forward by Dr Preetha Reddy, Dr Suneeta Reddy, Dr Shobana Kamineni and Dr Sangita Reddy who have propelled the Apollo Hospital Group to its position as the undisputed leader in healthcare in Asia.

The liver transplant program is indebted to the immense support from the Apollo Delhi management, our admission staff who have prioritized our critical patients, the billing and finance department that have allowed lifesaving emergency surgeries on credit when funds were not ready, our blood bank, emergency staff, microbiology, lab services, histopathology, radiologists, anesthetists, intensivists and pediatric super specialties, junior medical staff, paramedics and nurses, physiotherapists, and pharmacists (who constantly work long hours).

We are constantly in awe of our transplant surgeons who seem to always be in the hospital in scrubs—sacrificing holidays, weekends, festivals and many a time special family occasions and milestones in their prime years—working tirelessly to make excellent outcomes possible. A big salute to them, blessed are they to be chosen, for these roles.

We are grateful to Mr P Shivakumar, Mr CP Tyagi, Dr Bipin Puri and Dr Gaurav Katyal for their support.

We are what our families make us. Our parents, who nurture us, educate us, give us good values; and our partners and children, who give us the energy and motivation to go on in this daunting and draining mission, console us in our losses and rejoice in our victories, give us confidence when it begins to shake, and, most of all, spare the long golden hours that were entitled to be theirs … no words can thank them enough. We would like to express our gratitude to Sanjeev, Kunal, Manav, Nandini, Devaang and Tanya for their understanding.

Thank you to all our patients and their families for their trust. It takes a lot of courage to put through two of your nearest ones through major surgeries and especially the fit and healthy donor. We thank them for their faith in modern medicine.

We would like to thank Rakesh and Krishita from Harper Collins for taking up this assignment.

BIBLIOGRAPHY

1. Lorenzo D'Antiga. Pediatric Hepatology and Liver Transplantation. Springer Nature Switzerland AG 2019
2. Frederick J. Suchy et al. Liver Disease in Children. 5th edition. Cambridge medicine 2021
3. Kleinman et al. Walker's Pediatric Gastrointestinal Disease. 6th edition. People's medical Publishing House-USA Raleigh, North Carolina. 2018
4. Guandalini S et al. Textbook of Pediatric Gastroenterology, Hepatology and Nutrition. Springer International Publishing Switzerland 2016
5. Kleigman et al. Nelson Textbook of Pediatrics. 22nd edition Elseiver.
6. Poonacha P, Sibal A, Soin AS, Rajashekar MR, Rajakumari DV. India's first successful pediatric liver transplant. Indian Pediatr. 2001;38:287-91

7. Sibal A, Bhatia V, Gupta S. Fifteen years of liver transplantation in India. Indian Pediatr. 2013;50:999-1000

8. Sibal A, Malhotra S, Guru FR, Bhatia V, Kapoor A, Seth S, Jerath N, Jasuja S, Rajkumari V, Wadhawan M, Aggarwal DK, Guleria S, Shrivastava RN, Gupta S. Experience of 100 solid organ transplants over a five-yr period from the first successful pediatric multi-organ transplant program in India. Pediatr Transplant. 2014 Nov;18(7):740-5. doi: 10.1111/petr.12324. Epub 2014 Aug 4. PMID: 25092050

9. Malhotra S, Sibal A, Bhatia V, Kapoor A, Gopalan S, Seth S, Jerath N, Wadhawan M, Gupta S. Living Related Liver Transplantation for Biliary Atresia in the Last 5 years: Experience from the First Liver Transplant Program in India. Indian J Pediatr. 2015 Oct;82(10):884-9. doi: 10.1007/s12098-014-1687-x. Epub 2015 Feb 25. PMID: 2570805

10. Malhotra S, Sibal A, Goyal N. Pediatric Liver Transplantation in India: 22 Years and Counting. Indian Pediatr. 2020 Dec 15;57(12):1110-1113. PMID: 33318322

11. Jain S, Kumar K, Malhotra S, Venuthurimilli A, Goyal N, Sibal A. Understanding the living-related pediatric liver transplantation donor's decision process: A questionnaire-based retrospective study. J Pediatr Gastroenterol Nutr. 2024 Feb 1. doi: 10.1002/jpn3.12145. Epub ahead of print. PMID: 38299260.

12. Malhotra S, Sibal A. Emerging socioeconomic trends in pediatric liver transplantation in India. Indian Pediatr.2022;59(12):959

13. Agrawal S, Kumar K, Malhotra S, Venthurimilli A, Goyal N, Sibal A. Liver transplantation in Crigler-Najjar Syndrome Type I: A single center experience. Journal of clinical and experimental hepatology. Vol 12, 2S60-S61. 2022. DOI: 10.1016/j.jceh.2022.07.153

14. B Sahoo, K Kumar, S Agrawal, Y Jebaying, S Malhotra, A K Venuthurimilli, N Goyal, A Sibal. Pre and Per-liver transplant clinical course and outcome of children diagnosed as biliary atresia in the context of accompanying cystic changes in biliary tree-A comparative study. Journal of Clinical and Experimental Hepatology. Vol 13, S145, 2023. DOI:https://doi.org/10.1016/j.jceh.2023.07.214.

ABOUT THE AUTHORS

Dr Smita Malhotra is senior consultant, pediatric gastroenterology and hepatology at Indraprastha Apollo Hospital, Delhi. She has a special interest in pediatric liver transplantation and is actively involved in the pre/postoperative care of children undergoing liver transplantation and in their long term follow up.

She has dedicated her career to providing exceptionally daunting and challenging healthcare services to children with liver and gastrointestinal diseases. She is an accomplished orator and has spoken at several esteemed platforms to share her experience. She holds multiple prestigious research publications and book chapters to her credit.

Prof. Anupam Sibal set up the pediatric gastroenterology and hepatology unit at Indraprastha Apollo Hospital, Delhi in 1997, the first in the private sector in India. He helped establish the first successful liver transplant program in India in 1998. Prof. Sibal has been serving as Group Medical Director, Apollo Group since 2005.

Prof. Sibal served as President, Global Association of Physicians of Indian Origin (GAPIO) from 2020-22 and member of Institute Body, PGIMER Chandigarh from 2009-2014.

He has edited a textbook in Pediatric Gastroenterology and Hepatology and Nutrition. He has, to his credit, 165 publications, sixteen chapters, more than 400 National and International lectures.

Dr Sibal is the author of the National best seller *Is Your Child Ready to face the World?*

HarperCollins *Publishers* India

At HarperCollins India, we believe in telling the best stories and finding the widest readership for our books in every format possible. We started publishing in 1992; a great deal has changed since then, but what has remained constant is the passion with which our authors write their books, the love with which readers receive them, and the sheer joy and excitement that we as publishers feel in being a part of the publishing process.

Over the years, we've had the pleasure of publishing some of the finest writing from the subcontinent and around the world, including several award-winning titles and some of the biggest bestsellers in India's publishing history. But nothing has meant more to us than the fact that millions of people have read the books we published, and that somewhere, a book of ours might have made a difference.

As we look to the future, we go back to that one word—a word which has been a driving force for us all these years.

Read.